ISBN: 979-8-9877706-2-7

# Disclosure

I, the author, am not certified or licensed in any way, shape, or form to give professional advice on sexual or relationship matters. Nor am I a professional wrestler. This is a passion piece of literature rather than a professional one. By reading further you hold me unaccountable to anything that may or may not happen to you regarding headscissors. Do as you will with this information.

# This Book is Dedicated to…

My lover. I want to thank you for all the love filled headscissoring I selfishly require from you. Even if you dislike it, maybe dedicating a whole book in your honor will make it up to you. Sex is the biggest way I feel loved, and I appreciate your understanding of my needs on a level I myself don't even understand. Regardless, I hope this dedication makes you feel the way I feel when you willingly and lovingly scoop me up into your headscissors. Thank you for everything you do and are.

# Table of Contents:

# Introduction

You may have encountered individuals expressing a keen interest in experiencing a woman squeezing their head with her thighs. At first glance, these propositions and desires might have appeared unsettling, crude, or even morally objectionable to you. However, if your partner has insisted you to read this book with urgency similar to a matter of life and death, or if you've found yourself intrigued by the idea of getting your neck and head squeezed by a woman's legs, this book is designed to offer clarity.

Within these pages, you'll find answers to most questions you may have regarding the act of headscissoring. Whether you seek to understand the various types and intensities of headscissoring, desire to improve connection and intimacy with your partner, wish to comprehend your partner's desires, or aim to explore your own, this book is here to provide guidance. My goal is to equip you with the initial knowledge and resources needed to navigate this aspect of intimacy and potentially fulfill these desires for you or your partner.

Without further ado, I present to you:

# Headscissors

## The Guide to Satisfaction

Written by: K.O. Quinnvale

# Chapter 1

## What and Who

The first thing that typically pops into somebody's mind when they hear headscissors is, "What?" The next response after further explanation for the sexual sense tends to be, "Wait…what?" To answer the 'what' in its entirety, **headscissoring is an act of intimacy where one partner (the submissive) lets their head, neck, or face be tucked tightly between the thighs, calves, or legs of the other partner (the dominant)**. From here the dominant applies pressure to the submissive by squeezing firmly or stretching their legs outwards. For the sake of simplicity we will also encompass all types of bodyscissors within the headscissors category from now on, and a bodyscissor is where any part of the submissive's body (typically the torso, waist, or arms) gets squeezed by the dominant's legs in the same manner as a headscissor.

Using the terms submissive and dominant can also raise more questions, and while one partner tends to be dominant and the other tends to be submissive that doesn't necessarily mean headscissoring is an extremely kinky or taboo sexual act. To further elaborate on headscissoring, it is an act of intimacy which allows two partners to experience strength and closeness in a way that they never have before. It quite literally is an art that one can learn over time…a craft to be perfected to the liking of two individuals partaking in the intimate act. Being caught, squeezed, and trapped between someone's legs or catching, squeezing, and trapping someone between your own legs is the most basic and simple imagery of headscissoring in the sexual sense I can provide.

A very common response to the definition of a headscissor in the intimate and sexual context (what this book is all about) is, "I've never heard of that before, who the hell actually does that to people? Who would even want to have that happen to them?" These simple yet valid questions lead us to our 'Who?'. While the 'who' can vary greatly, there definitely is a trend and majority when it comes to gender and desire for this act of intimacy. The 'who' is men. Men are the most likely to desire or enjoy being headscissored whereas women are more likely to enjoy or desire doing the headscissors. Obviously, the data on this is very scarce and the 'who' does not have a sturdy and concrete answer at this point in time nor is it backed by solid sources. Based on my miniscule sample size of less than one-hundred, men want to be headscissored more than women. In addition, online pornographic content seems to lean this way in the sense that there is more content for this specific dynamic. It is also my hypothesis that the men want the women to headscissor them more than the women want to headscissor the men. As expected, there will always be outliers to this where a woman may desire headscissoring her partner to begin with, or where a man may not want to be headscissored at all. This is perfectly fine, as is any combination of genders or desires. Headscissoring is not for everybody in the world, and this book is merely here to help those who **_are_** interested in learning more about it whether they have the desire or not.

Anyways, as stated prior, when lurking through the internet for pornographic content on headscissoring the vast majority of results include men getting headscissored by women. This only reinforces my belief that men want to be headscissored by women the most. However, men are the largest target audience for porn, so the volume of headscissor pornography that exists doesn't necessarily reflect the female desire on this subject. Unsurprisingly, the second largest pornographic-content result was women getting headscissored by women. All other combinations of headscissors were miniscule in results, but their existence and desire by the minority of people who may enjoy them should never be discounted.

As I said, the last thing I want to do is discount the validity and desire to have any combination of genders in a headscissor. Anyone can be headscissored or get headscissored by anyone else assuming consent is on the table. With that being said though, the majority of available porn has men getting headscissored by women. Therefore the male < female combination is what the rest of this book will focus on. Nearly nothing changes in the types of headscissor, degree of headscissor, reasons for headscissoring, etc. The only thing changing will be the grammar and verbiage I use moving forward. Anyone can partake in headscissors, but a majority of this book will be written with the understanding that you are either a man wanting to be headscissored by a woman or a woman wanting to headscissor a man. Thank you for understanding.

So the logical next question one may have would be, "What is wrong with these men? Why in the world would they ever want to be headscissored by a woman? Why would a woman actually want to headscissor a man?" While there is nothing inherently wrong with any of the men who want to be headscissored, it is still important to ask them why they want to be headscissored. The 'what' and 'who' of headscissoring is generally blunt and simple, already answered in a couple paragraphs. However, the 'why' of headscissoring opens up lots of doors and helps one better understand their partner's or their own desires for such an intense act of intimacy.

# Chapter 2

## Why

Why do men want this? Do people actually enjoy it? Why would a woman want to do this to a man? The origination of sexual desires in an individual can be attributed to anything and everything including biological factors, psychological factors, and social factors. By no means am I certified to do an in depth analysis of even one of those factors. Instead, I will provide some of the surface level reasons somebody may be interested in the specific act of headscissoring. A lot of these reasons may only raise more questions about one's sexuality and who they really are at their core.

This may sound discouraging because you got this book for answers, and the answers I provide very well may only raise harder and deeper questions which can't be answered by the contents in this book. That is what it feels like to grow. You may learn why you like headscissors, but the truth behind it may require more extensive research to unravel deeper mysteries you may or may not have. With that being said, we will start by answering the 'why' for men. Then we will briefly look into the 'why' for the ladies too.

The first group of reasons a man may be interested or find enjoyment in headscissoring can be referred to as simple sensations. Firstly within that group we have **fixated arousal**. Crurophila can be defined as the love of or erotic fixation of legs. When somebody essentially has an obsession with a body part such as the legs, any sexual act where they get to be as close as possible to them will provide obvious satisfaction. This can happen in the form of smothering, rubbing, kissing, squeezing, stroking, or even headscissoring. The sexual attraction towards the legs is a very simple reason someone may enjoy being headscissored, and if instead it is a sexual obsession of the legs, crurophilia, that merely makes the passionate desire burn brighter.

Then there is **closeness**. This is another simple reason that doesn't necessarily have anything to do with arousal. This is just when the man enjoys the closeness he feels when trapped in his partner's headscissor. They feel close, warm, and loved since they are literally close, warm, and by the nature of headscissors, forced to cuddle closely to their partner's private parts. If a man enjoys being headscissored for this reason they may view the act more as intense and forced cuddling instead of a wrestling hold or sexual itch that needs scratching.

Simple arousal also includes **ass**. Yes, it really is that simple and that arousing. In some headscissor types or positions the female's ass may take up most of the male's field of vision. Men, being visual creatures, typically would never have a problem with their beloved partner displaying their beauty for them, let alone forcing them to witness their beauty up close and personal. Coupled with other acts of intimacy such as kissing or rubbing, this is perhaps the easiest reason to understand why a man might want to get headscissored by a woman.

The last reason subsiding in the simple arousal category is the **physicality** of the headscissor itself. Sometimes it just feels amazing to get squeezed out a little bit. Believe it or not, some men just enjoy the way that headscissoring feels. Whether it is the pain, the softness of a woman's legs on their neck and head, or the warmth of the hold it just feels good to experience without any sexuality needing to be attached to it.

Not all reasons are black and white though. The next category of reasons involves some sort of underlying kink. The very first thing that comes to my mind is femdom. **Femdom** is a sexual kink where women dominate men. This clearly plays on sexual polarity in the bedroom. While most men, at their core, want to sexually dominate, many men still desperately need to be sexually dominated by a woman. Nothing is wrong with that. The only problem is that women, for a majority, are the inverse. Meaning, most women want to be sexually dominated. The femdom kink typically is more intense than just dominant and submissive polarity. If a man enjoys headscissors because he is into femdom then chances are he also enjoys it when women dominate, belittle, and make him feel as though he is less than his female counterpart if not subservient or enslaved to her. This can be sexual in nature or even extend out of the bedroom. It also can be soft femdom or hardcore femdom, the difference being how brutal and intense the form of domination is.

The next underlying kink is **humiliation**. Much simpler than femdom, humiliation is where the man enjoys being physically overpowered and emasculated by a woman. While there are definitely aspects of that present in femdom, humiliation on its own typically is less brutal and only exists to make the man feel like he is a loser or unworthy, not that he is enslaved to a woman. They are very similar but slightly different.

Following humiliation is **masochism**. Masochism is defined as the tendency to derive sexual gratification from one's own pain or humiliation. Obviously, it is similar to humiliation, but it focuses more on the physically painful aspects. Here the man simply enjoys being hurt. They like the way the pain turns them on, and typically they also want a woman to provide it. Headscissors are an easy answer that fulfills their needs perfectly.

The last category of reasons a man may enjoy or desire headscissoring has some overlap from the previous categories. The first and most transparent desire for headscissors is **submission**. The man simply wants to submit sexually to his woman. Some may argue that literally any and every time he ejaculates he submits to the woman. True or false, he doesn't want to pretend to be in control until that point. He wants to submit long before the finish line. Why would the male want to be submissive? As I said before, most men don't, but a lot of them still want to. There are billions of people and millions of men who want to be submissive. Again, why do they want to be submissive? That is a loaded question that I can't answer to completion. However, I can give a couple ideas.

Firstly, they may be dominant every hour of their waking life, making every decision at work or constantly in control. They may need something to balance out their day, and sex could be a great option.

Second, they may want to feel free. Sexual submission is blissful indeed, so who is to deny them the relief of slipping under the control of another who confidently leads them to sexual satisfaction? Lastly, it may just be part of who they are. They might be sexually submissive at their core. This doesn't necessarily mean that they are homosexual, a woman inside a man's body, or into butt stuff. It just means that they get more sexual satisfaction from submitting rather than dominating. However, they still can be capable of both submitting and dominating, and they might even enjoy it.

Another polarity related reason men enjoy headscissoring is something I like to call **forced love**. Submissive in nature, headscissoring forces the man to be close to the woman's genitals. Whether the woman simply keeps him trapped, squeezes him dizzy, or sexually stimulates him further while in the headscissor, the man has no control. He is forced to experience his partner's love. No longer must he fight the world, for once she catches him it's all over. He can give in. He has been conquered. The outcome of the sexual act is no longer in his control, and this can provide an extreme and incomparable sense of freedom, especially if he tries to escape and is prevented.

While the previous two reasons blur slightly together, the last one blurs the most by being the simplest and arguably the most wholesome reason a man might enjoy headscissors. This reason is **love**. It is at this point you may need to rethink how you describe submissiveness. Perhaps you view it simply as the partner on the bottom. Maybe you think of it as the partner with no control, and to that I agree, to an extent. You may even think of submissive as the partner who gives oral, and that is easily wrong, also to an extent. When it comes to headscissoring however, a strong positive aspect of submissiveness is not necessarily just to be controlled, rather the desire to sacrifice your own strength to serve your lover. Furthermore, submissiveness doesn't always mean weakness or obedience. It is more about having your own strength and willingly relinquishing it to your partner. Meaning, dominance is less about controlling or exploiting your partner and more about leading them while enjoying the control over them that they desire to cede to you.

Enough of that though, let's get to the point. The main concept here is that the man wants to build trust with their partner by consciously forfeiting control and putting themselves in an extremely submissive position. Mainly to allow their partner to be as strong and feminine as she possibly can be, give her that sense of intoxicating power over him. They want to let their woman experience and feel her own strength in a way that she probably never has before. That alone is satisfaction for them, but since she is practicing on them, they get the best seat in the house to experience their lover learning of and enjoying her own strength first hand. Who doesn't want to watch their loved one learn and enjoy their own strength? Who doesn't want to be the exact reason that their loved one got to learn and enjoy their own strength in a manner most likely foreign to them? In my opinion this reasoning behind the desire for headscissors is one of if not the best reasons hands down. Also, out of love, they may enjoy headscissors, *simply because you do.*

Now, I know that there are probably more reasons men enjoy being headscissored. This book by no means is conclusive. With headscissoring as a whole being very untalked of there is still much to learn. Not to mention, the understanding of sexual desire to begin with is arguably still in its infancy. It also should go without saying that why somebody might like headscissors isn't exclusive to one of the reasons listed above. Somebody may have several conflicting reasons they enjoy headscissors. This only makes them more of a unique individual. I have polled a few about their own desires on the topic and would like to share the results with you. For further insight, here are some real life testimonials (well…Reddit testimonials…I know…data is scarce on this subject) answering the question: What is the #1 reason you enjoy headscissors?

"I'm a big leg man ever since I was a teenager and loved dominant women and I stumbled across headscissors and mixed wrestling when I was 14 and was hooked ever since and then…I discovered knockouts and oh god that was the cherry on the cake." ---Dom-Colour

"I'd say feeling her thigh muscles explode when they are flexed and squeezing me…seeing the passion and anger in her face while she is breaking me with her muscular legs…The feeling of the power of her muscular legs when she is squeezing. Also She's naturally a little on the shy side, so seeing a whole different side of her when She enjoys punishing me knowing how strong her legs are." ---Competitive-Grade887

"When I got headscissored there surprisingly wasn't a sexual turn on, but the squeeze of their thighs just felt good for some reason." ---Most_Progress9242

"For me, combo of the squeeze / choke sensation, the feeling of being trapped, but also the placement. I love thighs and ass lol." ---FancySouth8327

"The feeling of being dominated honestly." ---Okidiot11111

"For me, it's the feeling of being overpowered and trapped , not being able to do anything but staring at your captor while they're knocking you out." ---Ok-Sherbet2237

"I think it is that the thought of my face which is covered in freckles gets squished and red, then she teases me about it." ---Vast-Guess-4153

As you can see, lots of these self proclaimed interests contain more than just one of the reasons I listed in greater detail. If you are a man or love a man dearly, please take the time to go through all of the reasons one may enjoy headscissoring and try to decide which ones you or your partner personally may or may not have. If you are a woman or love a woman dearly, please take the time to continue reading and try to decide which reasons you or your partner may or may not have.

For the females, I will go in much less detail (sorry data is even more scarce for you), but I will still hit a few different reasons that I personally believe could exist. First and foremost, **strength** comes to my mind. Some women may enjoy headscissoring men for the simple fact that they want to feel strong and overpower another. Realizing you have the strength to put a man to sleep, despite him being seven feet tall and two hundred and fifty pounds, is quite the confidence boost. Next up we have **sadism**. This is the opposite of masochism. Here sexual gratification is derived from hurting or watching others experience physical or emotional pain.

Another reason, that men rarely have the privilege of experiencing, is **business**. Some women don't actually enjoy headscissors directly, but they enjoy the money they make from headscissoring. This can include, pornstars, session girls, content creators, or women of the night.

Just like the men who enjoy submitting, there are women who enjoy **dominating**. They simply enjoy being in control of their partner physically and sexually in a way that can also please their partner and themselves physically and sexually. Also, women can enjoy the powerful **love** reason. They too might want to showcase to their partner how powerful and strong their legs are by means of headscissoring, or they may enjoy the act of intimacy simply because their partner likes it. They can even build sexual polarity by headscissoring as well as fostering trust in their partners by giving a good headscissor session. Lastly, like men it can all boil down to **simple arousal** or **closeness**. Having their partner trapped right next to their genitals might make a woman feel warm and cozy and for good reason. Sometimes just squeezing something tightly with their legs can outright make them feel good. Even if it happens to be a man's head.

Now, just as I did for the men's reasons, I will provide a Reddit testimonial from a potential woman who might enjoy headscissoring, answering why they enjoy it:


"Money. Oh, and the other reason is money." ---Deleted Account

At the time of writing this, that was the single response that was submitted from a community of over twenty-five thousand people. The comment was deleted along with the account shortly after it was posted. Chances are it might not have even been a woman who said it. As I said before, there is a major lack of data for this sexual desire that men have. Therefore, finding concrete facts or even self reported opinions about women's desires around this topic is even more difficult and inconclusive. I'm positive some women genuinely enjoy headscissoring and for great reasons. I am also positive I've missed a plethora of reasons, but for now this can act as a guide to help you brainstorm your true reasons for enjoying headscissors. If that is something you do happen to like.

# Chapter 3

## The Degrees and Dynamics of Headscissors

Not all headscissors are the same because each hold or positioning can bring different sensations to both partners. We will talk more about the different holds or techniques in a later chapter. In this chapter we focus more on the intensity of the headscissor session. A headscissor session being an extended period of time where headscissors occur. The exact time can vary greatly, but as a guide for satisfaction a session should be around a minimum of five minutes long. Otherwise, it can feel unfulfilling and rushed. A degree is best applied to a headscissor session, and to help you understand, equate each degree as the intensity rating for the headscissor session in question.

Here are the following degrees to headscissoring:

**Zero Degree Headscissor.** A zero degree headscissor is simply anything but a headscissor. It is walking through the park. It is sitting on the bus. It is hugging your grandma. Consider this degree the normal resting state absent of any headscissors. Like stage one dementia, we all have experienced this degree but forget it even exists. Let's keep it that way.

**First Degree Headscissor.** The first degree headscissor is much more relaxed than one might imagine. It is where the man's head (or body) is between the woman's legs. No squeezing is required. The only requirement is that <u>the woman's legs are around the man</u>. Examples of this can include, cunnilingus, cuddling where thighs are thrown over or coiled around the man's waist, piggy back rides, and even the cowgirl sex position where she straddles his torso. The woman's legs don't even have to be touching the man for it to fall into this category.

**Second Degree Headscissor**. The second degree headscissor adds intentional physical contact. No longer is the man simply between a pair of legs. Here the legs must be somewhat constricted around the man. That is the only difference. The legs must be coiled around and pressed against the man. The woman can squeeze softly if she chooses, but that isn't required or frequent. Extremely similar to the first degree, the required contact now brings her legs slightly into more focus. Here the male gets to be intimately close to the female without any form of dominant or submissive polarity. The man can escape at will if he pleases, and the legs never lock to prevent any escape attempts. Jiggling of the ass can happen as a form of teasing.

**Third Degree Headscissor**. The third degree introduces helplessness. Building on the second degree where the legs must be touching the man, now escaping the woman's legs is no longer an option. In a third degree headscissor, if the male attempts to escape (without using the established safe word) the female prevents it with all her strength. Still, squeezing can happen, but it isn't a main feature of the degree or used too frequently. However, if the man attempts to escape, the woman can squeeze as much as she desires to punish him. The pressure should equal the strength of the escape attempt, but as you will learn this can vary based on the dynamic. Quite literally, the man will get what he asks for unless he obeys and remains content between the woman's legs.

**Fourth Degree Headscissor**. In the fourth degree squeezing and applying of pressure occurs frequently. Of course, as we continue up in degrees everything established previously is built upon. Therefore, the male still is not capable/allowed to escape the headscissor, but now the female frequently applies pressure even when the man isn't attempting to escape. At this stage, she doesn't hold any squeeze long enough to make him submit, and she never squeezes as hard as she can. After every squeeze, depending on the dynamic, a grace period can follow. Soft, pulsing squeezes where the female squeezes quickly in rapid fire contractions can be exploited here, but these should be soft and generous because the male should never need to tap out in a fourth degree headscissor. (A tap out is a physical gesture made by the male which communicates his submission and inability to continue the current hold.)

**Fifth Degree Headscissor**. Caught in a fifth degree headscissor? You are going to tap out. In the fifth degree at some point the male submits, typically by tapping out. The main difference between the previous stage and this one is that <u>the male consciously submits</u>. The female squeezes harder and longer. The man can tap out once or one hundred times in this stage, but the female still provides the assurance that he won't be knocked unconscious. When he taps, she usually will release pressure depending on the dynamic, but even in dynamics where his taps are religiously disobeyed she makes sure he never passes out. She might give him grace periods between tap outs. Still, she shouldn't have to squeeze him with all her strength.

**Sixth Degree Headscissor**. With a sixth degree headscissor things change drastically. The first and most notable point is that <u>the female headscissors the male to the point he passes out, completely ignoring the male's taps</u>. The instant he is knocked out is typically the telltale sign the headscissor session has changed from the fifth to the sixth degree. In the sixth degree however, the male is only knocked unconscious once. After that point it is the woman's job to ensure he doesn't pass out again, especially if the dynamic prevents tap outs.

**Seventh Degree Headscissor**. At the second consecutive knockout, one may find themself in a seventh degree headscissor session. <u>The male is knocked out for the second time, and all taps are ignored, mocked, or even prevented completely</u>. There is no limit to the amount of knockouts that can occur in the seventh degree, and regardless of the dynamic there is no limit to what the female is allowed to do when it comes to squeeze pressure, squeeze length, and grace periods with the exception that once knocked out, squeezing must stop. After getting to the seventh degree, the man must be aware that at any time the woman can put him to sleep. This can create senses of unpredictability and fear for him and senses of power and control for her.

**Eighth Degree Headscissor**. Few have ventured this far. Unfortunately, in the eighth degree the risks heavily outweigh the rewards. The only difference here is that after the male is knocked out, the female can keep squeezing. <u>No longer does the woman have to follow any form of safety protocol, mainly squeeze length after a knockout. Visible injury of the male typically occurs at some capacity</u>. This can result in vomiting, brain damage, nosebleeds, stroke, changes in blood pressure, etc. It is highly encouraged to avoid this degree of headscissoring for your partner's and your own safety, but two consenting adults can decide to do whatever they wish to do with one another.

**Ninth Degree Headscissor**. The headscissor of fiction. While I 100% advise against attempting all eighth degree headscissors let alone a ninth degree, the ninth degree is the highest degree of headscissors. Unlike the eighth degree, the female continues to squeeze after the male is knocked unconscious, not for a short time either, but until he passes. Correct, you read that right, a ninth degree headscissor is defined by the death of the male. Yes, <u>the woman literally kills the man with her legs</u>. While it can be erotic and hot to witness animations of a male being squeezed to death by a nice pair of thighs, do not attempt this in real life. Some men may agree it is the best way to die or even make jokes about wanting this exact thing, but it is dying nonetheless. Once dead, there may or may not be any more headscissors to find yourself caught in. Steer clear of the ninth degree and let fiction have the monopoly on this one.

**Null Degree Headscissor**. The null degree or unknown degree is a special degree that can transcend other degrees. An null degree headscissor can exist in the eighth degree or the first. The thing that defines this degree is the male's acceptance of uncertainty and total submission. Typically, a couple might discuss and decide together what the highest degree headscissor they are going to try in a specific session, but in this case the male relinquishes the right to know that going into the session. Of course, the couple can and should agree, for example, that they will not go past the sixth degree, but the man still doesn't know if the woman will bring him to the sixth or only to the third degree. This option exists to give the woman more control over the man. She chooses whether or not the man will be knocked out, and he has no knowledge about the degree of headscissoring he will find himself in until it happens. This can also be beneficial for couples who have scissored for a while. The woman knows what the man is capable of handling, and this degree adds the pleasure of swiftness and unpredictability. If the man is curious and asks her what degree she plans on taking him to, she is not obligated to tell him. I will talk more about practical uses of this degree in a later chapter.

After learning all the fun concepts and new ways of perceiving a headscissor session, the degrees can be enhanced for more pleasure if the two parties understand why they enjoy headscissors. Hence the importance of the previous chapter. The reason someone enjoys headscissors and the personality/actions of the female and male during a session can affect how certain degrees feel for the male and how much enjoyment the female gets. For example, with a man who enjoys headscissors strictly because of love, a third degree headscissor where the female simply holds him there and hugs him may feel much more rewarding when compared to a eighth degree headscissor where the female belittles him verbally and gets off on his visible pain.

Another example is where a woman who enjoys being dominant and overpowering likes it more when the man squirms and tries to escape rather than when the man is motionless and accepts his fate between her legs. It is also important to note that some people enjoy higher degrees over lower ones and other people enjoy lower degrees over higher ones. There is nothing wrong with what degree you or your partner like the most. Also, as time passes it is expected that your own desires might change. Thus, the highest degree you or your partner would ever consider experiencing could change over time.

This is why in addition to the degrees or intensities of a headscissor session, we can also attach a specific dynamic to a session. As mentioned before, certain dynamics can change how a degree feels or is executed, and these dynamics can illustrate the reasons why somebody enjoys headscissoring to begin with. Dynamics can change how the parties in a headscissor session move, behave, communicate, appear, and how they interpret the degrees to best fulfill their reasons for enjoying headscissors. However, the dynamics are different than the degrees because they can be much more loosely followed to the point where a dynamic isn't existent in a particular session at all.

Learning Dynamic. The learning dynamic is typically the first dynamic a couple uses when trying headscissoring for the first time. It is not common to find videos of this dynamic online because it is a slow and communicative form of headscissoring where the woman allows both herself and her man to learn and experience the sensations for possibly the first time. This dynamic follows the degree classification loosely and typically occurs in the fifth degree or lower. Tap outs are immediately obeyed unless in a sixth degree or higher, and the woman is constantly taking time to ensure the man is comfortable, conscious, and enjoying the experience. Simultaneously, she is learning more about her own body by realizing which holds her man prefers, which holds he submits to the quickest, and which holds feel the best for her. It doesn't matter if both of the partners have experience headscissoring, this dynamic can still work wonders for building trust and deepening understanding of each other's bodies.

Relaxed Dynamic. The relaxed dynamic is quite similar to the learning dynamic, but instead of taking time to learn the couple takes time to be close. Taps are usually obeyed unless a knockout is desired, and there isn't much teasing or verbal communication related to the headscissor session itself. The partners can rub, kiss, massage, and squeeze each other, or they can focus on something unrelated to them completely, such as a movie or a book. They can take this time together to talk about their day or anything else on their minds. The headscissor session itself doubles as cuddling and takes a backseat to whatever the couple wants to place more attention on in this dynamic.

Playful Dynamic. The playful dynamic adds truckloads of teasing to the session. The teasing is heavily verbal, but it is common to see the woman playing with the man's face or hair while scissoring him. It also is common to see her toying with him using her legs too. Grace periods are used a lot with this dynamic due to the increased verbal teasing. The man typically doesn't know when the woman will squeeze him because she keeps him trapped between her legs in a grace period for extended moments of time. An example of some teasing that might happen includes the woman suggesting just how powerful she feels before immediately squeezing tightly once the man attempts to respond to her. This dynamic is best used at the third degree or higher since the inescapable factor increases the playfulness. Knock outs aren't too important here as the woman wants the man to be able to hear her verbal charades. The playful dynamic is a great form of foreplay prior to other forms of sex which allows the woman to slip into a dominant and playful mindset.

**Polar Dynamic**. The polar dynamic furthers teasing down a specific path. Instead of teasing about what her thighs are going to do to him or how powerful she feels (although those can still be utilized) the focus is much more on the fact that she is his dominant and he is her submissive. The best degree to suit this dynamic is the fifth degree because grace periods aren't typically long when demonstrating her control over her man in a serious manner. Not only that, she wants to force her man to submit, maybe even beg for her to stop. Of course, she can still tease and play with him like the previous dynamic, but the focus now is much more on...well...dominating him. The woman doesn't care about letting the man learn how the different holds feel. She cares about making him laugh or learn. He is not in control, and her focus is satisfying not only herself but also him with the control he has relinquished to her. She only wants to dominate him to a point where he feels comfortable.

**Roleplay Dynamic**. The roleplay dynamic is very similar to the polar dynamic in the sense that there is a clear dominant and a clear submissive. However, instead of teasing about trivial and light hearted subjects like in the playful dynamic or the polarity of the situation like in the polar dynamic, there is a specific roleplay with specific ideas or outcomes that are referenced. This dynamic usually includes costumes, methods, and techniques that further engulf the parties into the roleplay (we will talk about methods and techniques in a later chapter). For example, let's look at a snake roleplay. Firstly this dynamic is different because the woman will be wearing a snake skin bodysuit or something similar to further the sense to everyone involved that she is a fierce predator. She will move slowly and seductively, putting her legs first and possibly even keeping close to the ground as if she were a snake. The man will reluctantly approach her or downright avoid her completely retreating from her advances. Eventually, the man will either allow her to coil her legs around his neck or get caught between her thighs against his will. Then she will slowly constrict her thighs around him. The whole time the two of them can be verbally teasing each other based on the nature of the roleplay at hand, the polarity dynamics, or whatever they want to tease about. This can be done with over a million different combinations of dominant and submissive ranging from categories such as snakes all the way to nurses. If you can think of it, you can roleplay it.

**Sadistic Dynamic**. The sadistic dynamic is a breed of its own. Yes, it can fall under the roleplay dynamic as can all other dynamics. However, like other dynamics independent of the roleplay dynamic there is something about it that makes it unique enough to have a category of its own. I like to look at this dynamic as the most extreme and intense form of headscissoring. Here the woman genuinely does not care about the man's physical health. She is consumed by her carnal desires and enjoys hurting him with headscissors. Most sessions of this dynamic end in the eight degree. The man usually has no point to tap out, is punished for it, or is completely restrained from attempting it to begin with. The satisfaction is one-hundred percent for the female, as the woman can and does push the man far beyond his limits every time simply for fun because she can. Hopefully he agreed and consented to the session prior because once it starts there is absolutely no safe word, and there is nothing the man can do to stop the session. This may sound just like any eighth degree headscissor session without a safe word, but the point here is that this dynamic exists purely in the eighth degree. There are no rules the woman must follow regarding the man's safety, and even if she provides a grace period it is understood that it is transitory at best. A good example I can provide if you want to see what I mean is a content creator named 'Lexi Long Legs'. I'm sure she has some free content, but don't say I didn't warn you.

# Chapter 4

## Options of fulfillment

Whether you are a man wanting a woman to headscissor you or a woman wanting to squeeze a man, there are multiple options to fulfill this sexual need. Not all ways to get headscissored are equal, and this book as a whole is definitely designed with one option in mind. However, whatever option you choose is valid for your own circumstances. Anyways, we will start by going over options of fulfillment for the men.

**Book a session**. While not the best long term solution, paying to have a session with a woman who regularly headscissors men for income is the easiest option. Chances are she will be a seasoned veteran of headscissoring and will dance around you with combos and positions you didn't know existed. Some of the session girls, as agreed upon by their terms, will knock you out repeatedly. Some of them are more generous and will only do so if you ask. You will be able to choose which woman you want (if she is available), and you can book a session where she will likely record herself absolutely dominating you for her online patrons. It is hard to build a loving or meaningful connection this way, but it can fulfill your needs if you are willing to pay the pricey fee and risk being on the internet for the rest of time.

**Pros:**
1. Easiest and safest.

2. Skilled headscissors.

3. You can pick whoever you want with ease.

4. Different girl each time.

5. Rare possibility to get a private video for yourself.

**Cons:**
1. Expensive.

2. May require traveling.

3. No connection (just another head for her to squeeze).

4. Empty fulfillment.

5. Potential lack of boundaries.

6. Possibility to be uploaded online.

**Find one night stands/women of the night**. This mainly focuses on creating a friends with benefits relationship where you call them up to fulfill this need once before ghosting them completely out of shame never to see them again. I'm just kidding. There is nothing to be ashamed of, but I know the majority of you would prefer your carnal desires be kept a secret. That's where friends with benefits come in. You can live your wildest dreams with them before breaking things off like they were never in your life to begin with, or better yet, see them occasionally for the good ole' squeeze session. Afterwards they return to their life, and nobody knows about your desires. Of course, while I don't recommend it due to the obvious legality conflict in some countries, this can be done with women of the night as well.

**Pros:**
1. Cheapest.

2. Boundaries.

3. No commitment/not online = nobody finds out about your headscissoring.

4. Convenient.

**Cons:**
1. Possibly illegal (if not FWB).

2. Unskilled headscissors.

3. Empty fulfillment.

4. Difficult to start FWB.

5. High risk being in such a submissive position with strangers.

**Get a girlfriend**. This is the most rewarding option for the fulfillment of your headscissor needs. Assuming she provides headscissors to fulfill your sexual needs, as all loving girlfriends do, she will learn which types, methods, and degrees you like, she will learn how to apply them faster, tighter, stronger, longer, she will learn how to make them inescapable yet equally desirable, and last but not least she might learn how to use them against you to get what she wants, occasionally. Sounds amazing right? There's a catch, and no it is not the "She headscissored me so she could pick what we watched on Netflix." No, that is the price we all willingly pay, but the following sequence is a much greater cost…Getting the girlfriend, convincing her to headscissor you, teaching her the types, degrees, and how to headscissor you, and managing to get continuously headscissored by her until your death by natural causes. Hats off to any man out there who successfully can complete that chain of events.

**Pros:**
1. Fulfilling Headscissors from your loving spouse.

2. Headscissor skills, methods, and techniques all perfected to conquer you.

3. Maximum trust, boundaries, and intimacy.

4. Connection and sexual polarity.

5. Maximum convenience.

6. Loving headscissors (she does it willingly to fulfill your needs, not because you pay her to or in exchange for sex).

7. Long term headscissors where she perfects her craft…on you…against you…in her holds…where she also learns your weaknesses. Similar to pro #2.

8. Surprise headscissors when least expected, sometimes to even take dominance outside the bedroom (can be a con if abused).

9. Possibility to get a private video for yourself.

**Cons:**
1. Maximum expense. While sessions cost hundreds per hour, a girlfriend costs much more than that, especially if you factor in emotional investment, mental energy, and stress.

2. Time investment. Excluding the financial expenses, it will take lots of time and practice for the two of you to learn the best way to partake in this highly intimate act.

3. Communicating. Sometimes, girlfriends are appalled by and opposed to headscissoring their beloved boyfriend for a plethora of reasons. Since you have this sexual need and since you have a girlfriend, chances are she is the only person in the world capable of fulfilling it for you. Marking this as a con if she refuses to headscissor you at all would be a great understatement. Using this book to help communicate this to her or decide if headscissors are truly a necessity for you would be a great idea.

4. Trust. You may not be at the level of trust required to safely partake in headscissors with your partner. Trusting that she keeps it confidential and doesn't use it against you in any manner is a hurdle not all overcome. A hurdle sometimes not meant to be overcome.

5. Rejection. If your loving partner is disgusted by your desire to be crushed between her thighs, that hurts. If she is unwilling to attempt to understand your desire or unwilling to fulfill it…that hurts even more.

6. Conquest. If you don't have a girlfriend you will need to get one. That is **NOT** an easy task for the vast majority of men.

7. Negative impact on the relationship. While not guaranteed, it is possible that your girlfriend will lose some respect for you when she watches your eyes glaze and daze and your mouth unconsciously drool in submission to the powerful, pulsing thigh muscles she conquered you with. The power trip may go to her head, especially if she does it to you unannounced all the time, and she may slip into a dominant role outside of the bedroom. This can turn into potential emasculation (not a con for some), and a flipping of the non-sexual polarity of the relationship can be detrimental if it was previously established. There is also a slim chance that if she sees you this way she may lose sexual attraction to you completely. This however is better to look at as a filter for your relationships because if anyone sees their partner weak and loses love and attraction for them…they probably didn't deserve the partner in the first place.

Now we will get into the options of fulfillment for the females out there that enjoy headscissoring for whatever reason that may be. Firstly, we have **sessions**. They could become a session girl who gets paid to headscissor strangers. While I advise against this, I must accept its place in our world. Sessions essentially are empty fulfillment devoid of strong love between the two parties. I am not saying there is anything wrong with sessions because of that. I am, however, advising that before getting into sessioning please take plenty of time to consider the pros and cons of being a sex worker in the first place. In addition to that, most session girls also create content for virtual consumption. It is advised that before sessioning to also consider the pros and cons for becoming a video girl or onlyfans girl, and you should consider how you will contribute to the porn industry. Regardless, I have a biased and major preference for session girls over girls who simply sell videos or photos because the session girls are providing the actual headscissor experience to a very few men who may not have ever had it otherwise. There is a demand for headscissors, and if you already have the desire to squeeze men between your legs for literally any reason, you can make some money here with relative ease.

**Pros:**
1. Money.

2. Chance at fame.

3. Empty fulfillment (you have no real intimate connection with the men).

4. Different victim each time.

5. You perfect your craft over time.

6. Power trip from men begging to be dominated by you.

**Cons:**
1. Considered a taboo career.

2. Possible objectification by your fans.

3. Contributing to the brain rot that is porn.

4. Power trip from men begging to be dominated by you.

5. Possible difficulty finding healthy intimate relationships.

6. Training required to be a session girl. Fit, attractive, gym, thick thighs, etc.

7. Start up can be initially disappointing and discouraging if your business grows too slowly.

Like men, we also have **parties/one night stands/being a woman of the night**. With the exception of the last one, all of these are legal in most countries, relatively easy to find, and low risk. While you may not like the suitors who approach you, strangers at that party, or whom you may be keeping in the friend zone, they do have a head nonetheless which means they are eligible to be squeezed. Depending on the reason you enjoy headscissoring this could validate them to be squeezed and become an easy way to fulfill your desire. In some rare cases, you may be able to headscissor your male friends and blow it off as a non-sexual act of superiority.

**Pros:**
1. Easiest, just ask a willing man to put his head between your legs.

2. Low risk, while offering sex to strangers or those you don't know fondly is extremely risky, if they are in your headscissor they are ultimately at your mercy.

3. Empty fulfillment.

4. Good practice.

5. New victims can be acquired.

**Cons:**
1. The victims can be undesirable at best.

2. May become known as the 'Headscissor Girl' locally.

3. Empty fulfillment, depending on your 'why' the lack of a connection may hurt you more in the long run, the same can be said for men who partake in empty fulfillment.

4. Lack of manly men. If every male friend you meet and get to know at one point submits and begs feverishly between your serpent-like, constricting thighs, your perception of men as a whole may be negatively impacted. Just remember, nobody is cool enough to catch a bullet and nobody is cool enough to escape a locked headscissor.

**Get a boyfriend**. Another option for you headscissor loving ladies is to simply communicate the fulfillment of your needs from your current or predicted boyfriend. While the men typically have to convince their partners, you simply have to show him. If he is a rare boyfriend who objects to a headscissor session with you, offer him fellatio in a strange position. If he agrees, scoop him up in a reverse headscissor of the third degree where you don't squeeze him. Go down on him, keep him there for a while, and if he still doesn't enjoy it then convincing and communicating your sexual needs more seriously may be required. Very rarely would a man not provide this if it is one of your top sexual needs and has been communicated properly.

**Pros:**
1. Fulfillment of your sexual need in the most loving way possible.

2. Connection, trust, boundaries, and intimacy.

3. You get to learn your man's weaknesses to your legs as you perfect your craft on him.

4. There is a high chance your boyfriend will want this from you or enjoy it anyways.

5. Convenience.

6. Possibility to double as cuddle time.

7. Inverted polarity. Typically the female is sexually submissive in the bedroom, so swapping roles can liven up the relationship and keep things fresh.

8. The 'Do what I say' look can end in a life draining reverse headscissor if your boyfriend fails to recognize and oblige to it (don't abuse it).

**Cons:**

1. Potential emasculation. Your boyfriend may feel weak, unrespected, and unfit to protect you if he slips unconscious between your man melters, damaging the relationship.

2. Power trip. You may find yourself unintentionally abusing your boyfriend with headscissors to get what you want in a non-sexual manner. While some guys will admit this is fine for trivial things on the infrequent occasion, this can be a serious problem if headscissors are used to dominate outside of the bedroom frequently.

3. Convincing. While rare you may have to spend some time convincing your boyfriend to let you headscissor him.

4. No boyfriend. If you currently don't have a boyfriend then acquiring one and building trust would be a hurdle to your headscissors.

5.  Unleashing the demon within. Whether it is you or your partner that learns they want headscissors much more frequently or intensely…this may be an unwelcome change for the relationship.

Notice that not once in the options for fulfillment did I mention porn. While I disagree with porn almost entirely, I understand its necessity for personal growth in some cases. I also understand that without it, headscissors wouldn't have ever crossed my mind, thus this book would never exist. It is very important for learning what you want sexually and new techniques to try in the bedroom. This combined with the fact that it can be consumed in a healthy manner prevents me from outright advising completely against it. The catch is the negative side effects from prolonged porn consumption, abuse, or addiction. Watching porn to fulfill your headscissor desires does not work completely due to the fact that it is the emptiest form of fulfillment. You will learn new techniques, dynamics, and methods of headscissoring that you didn't know you needed in your life, but it does not provide nearly the same satisfaction as the real deal. Just like normal porn doesn't remove your desire for sex. Headscissor porn likely will only make you want it more. It is a vicious cycle to find yourself caught in.

What about the creators who make headscissor content to help the public better understand their own desires? This is also equally important because if you only watch porn a couple of times to learn what you want before stopping (the ideal play) they would all go out of business. Even if you only watch free content they still will struggle financially and probably stop without the assistance of advertisements, but that is perfectly fine because the internet is now old enough to harbor plenty of content that will teach you all you didn't know.

This does not mean the content creators are useless, unneeded, or a waste of space or energy. They still deserve love and appreciation, and you can certainly provide that in the form of watch time or monetary donations. However, everybody knows the best content creators produce works of art because they have a passion for the subject, not because they want to make money. Do you think headscissoring content should be different? Regardless, what you spend your money on translates to your vote on what the world should have more of. In our modern times, what you spend time viewing or consuming also translates to your vote on what the world should have more of. By all means, you are entitled to cast your votes in whatever way you might want to.

There is another aspect of content creators that shouldn't be ignored...the sessions. Since sessions are in person and actual experiences that you could pay for, I would highly recommend them if the other options for fulfillment don't tickle your fancy. Onlyfans, Fansly, or paid content on the other hand...I will advise you not to pay for the potential empty fulfillment that free content could just as easily provide. If you want something uniquely specific, by all means pay for it to be created. Of course, you can send one of the creators money for the hard work they've done for the community, and that is encouraged. However, in my opinion, subscribing to an Onlyfans or Fansly is basically admitting defeat in your pursuit of real-life headscissors. Save that money and spend it to have a session with the same girl instead of buying her subscription. That way the creators still get paid for creating, and you get to experience real life headscissors by someone who gets paid to do them. Don't neglect the creators for putting themselves out there for us, but don't sacrifice everything you have to keep them in business, no matter how hot that may sound. (I am aware that sending all of your money to women online is an actual kink. I still would advise against that. Find a trusting and loving girl in real life to do that to. At least that way there is a higher chance she may have your best interest in mind.)

You may or may not agree with my take on paying for headscissor content. I am not suggesting you stop paying for content if you already are; this is rather a suggestion to avoid paying for content if you haven't done so in the past. You earn your money and deserve to spend it anywhere you wish. While at the surface level there is nothing wrong with subscribing to porn; lots of hidden problems have the risk to occur with even simple, unpaid porn consumption. However, if you take cautionary methods to prevent any of the negative side effects (body image issues, motivation, sexual dysfunction, depression, desire to isolate, porn addiction, unrealistic expectations, objectification, anxiety...) porn certainly can be the most empty form of fulfillment for your sexual needs. Porn has its place in our world, but my advice is to view it like a drug. Proceed with caution. Ultimately, for both genders, it is an option.

# Chapter 5

## Convincing your Partner

So you went out, got a girlfriend (or boyfriend), and hopefully have had sex at least a couple of times. You trust them enough to open up a little bit about your deeper sexual desires. You want to take the plunge and squirm in submission between their legs for whatever reason you may have. This is the final step between you and a long term headscissor fulfillment journey (assuming the relationship survives). It can almost be as nerve racking as getting them to be your partner in the first place. "What if they say no? What if they are disgusted and appalled? What if they say yes, but it is a horrible experience for us both? What if they say yes, but they secretly hate it?" These are all valid concerns one may have. This chapter will help you through all of this and more, and hopefully afterwards your partner may be convinced if at the very least to try headscissoring with you!

First and foremost you have to change the way you look at the whole equation. Convincing your girlfriend shouldn't be the goal, rather communicating your deepest sexual needs in a judgment free place with them. Your goal isn't to manipulate her into providing this sexual need for you, rather communicating it to her. Both of you must have an open mindset regarding sex in your relationship, open enough to at least listen to each other. In any relationship, having a partner who is closed and non-receptive to talking about sex can be bad. If she hasn't confided in you even the smallest detail about her sexually, chances are you're not in a sex-open relationship quite yet. She may be shy, she may be nervous, or she may be waiting for you to take the vulnerable leap where you open up about your sexuality. If that is the case it is very easy for you to break through this. In this particular case, just confide in her, "You have the most beautiful legs, and I would kiss them all night if I could."

This isn't too cheesy and lets her know you like her legs as well as being close to her legs. If she responds positively to this you can ask what she likes about you (remember relationships aren't all about you, so understanding their desires is equally important as conveying yours). Genuinely listen and plan to fulfill her desires in the future. Pay attention but don't let her get too carried away, before the discussion ends or changes, return the conversation to her legs and ask if at some point she would let you worship her inner thighs with kisses. If she says yes, congrats! While probably not the headscissor you want, you just scored yourself a first degree, possibly second degree headscissor! If she says no…you have lots of work to do before she can trust you or allow that. Ask her if at some point she would allow it. If the answer is still a no, the decision to nurse the relationship further rests in your hands as kissing her inner thighs is a very surface level sexual act.

Assuming she says yes, do exactly that at an appropriate time. While kissing away on her inner thighs you could easily tell her you like to be squeezed a little bit, and when she squeezes briefly give her a feral reaction. Immediately after she releases, attack her thighs with a thousand wet kisses. Go ballistic. Get in there. Go crazy. Show her that when she squeezes your head between her legs, you lose all control and lick her thighs like they came fresh from KFC and you're on a week long fast. What is she going to do? She will probably squeeze longer or tighter to see what you will do. Of course, you have to fulfill her expectations and up your kissing game if she does that, maybe even going for some soft cunnilingus before returning your attention to her thighs. Make it a game. A game where you calmly love on her legs until she squeezes you with them. If she squeezes, you aggressively love on her legs and even vulva. She will quickly learn the rules of the game: *If I lay here he kisses my thighs. If I squeeze him tightly between my thighs, upon release he passionately kisses my vulva for a few seconds before returning to my thighs*…It won't take long for her to exploit this and for you to find yourself in an inescapable cycle of soft headscissors and cunnilingus. Obviously, this is not long term, as eventually she will grow weary of the game and desire straight cunnilingus to relax into, and I advise you to provide her that when she desires it. However, this is enough to get your foot in the door, or your melon between her mashers to say.

If you have made it this far, chances are your partner will not deny headscissors of the first or second degree because of the positive experience you already gave them. The positive experience will open her mind to trying something like headscissoring especially when she realizes that she's already done it to you at a lower degree. At this point it is safe to simply say, "Hey my beloved [partner's name], I need to tell you something…[partner's response]...In the bedroom…I loved it when you headscissored me earlier, and I would like to take things further in that area."

Even playing all of these games is unnecessary. The point I am trying to make is just to be honest with them and show them it can be enjoyable for everyone involved. More likely than not if they love you enough they'd be willing to provide you with headscissors, after you explain what that is of course. What if they are disgusted by the concept? Explain to them that cunnilingus is considered a headscissor of the first and second degree. This may be a large generalization, but not too many women are turned off by cunnilingus. What if they remove cunnilingus entirely and are still disgusted by the act of headscissoring you? Ask them why. "Would headscissoring be disgusting if we both do it willingly and with love?"

Don't have this conversation before bed or after sex. If you are serious about this, which I assume you are since you're reading a book about it, have a serious discussion with your partner over food and at a good time. If they are disgusted, ask them why. Roleplay---rather be their therapist, and try to get to the root cause. They may just be saying it is gross because they think it is weird and unusual, but it isn't any more unusual when compared to deepthroating or anal. Both of which inherently are 'more disgusting' due to the fact that they are intercourse not outercourse.

What if they say yes, but it is a horrible experience for the both of you? Well…then headscissoring may not be something you necessarily desire as much as you thought. It may have been something you only thought you wanted. On the other hand, it may just be a sign that the two of you need more practice. Teach her what you like until you enjoy the experience, but let her do what she likes too. After all, she is the one in control here isn't she? Still, if headscissoring is such a taxing and deplorable experience for her, go down on her until she finishes twice for every one headscissor session. Be sure to pay upfront, that way she doesn't feel the urge to rush through the session. Furthermore, ask her what she would want you to do to her sexually to make up for a headscissoring session. If you are okay with doing that, do it. I am not trying to make your sex life transactional by any means, which is why I also advise you to not ask for a headscissor session afterwards. Communicate your desire to be headscissored but don't ask for it. Give her what she said she wanted in return for a headscissor session, SEVEN times before even asking once about your needs. By then she will probably have given you a session willingly after realizing your love for her triumphs over your own sexual needs. Sexual selflessness is key in this scenario. If she still doesn't offer it after six or seven times by all means begin communicating sexual needs from your lover. If she refuses, it is up to you whether or not you want to keep the relationship on life support.

What if my partner agrees to headscissor me but secretly hates it? First off, congratulations on being in their mind and knowing they secretly hate it. Secondly, congratulations on getting yourself some headscissors. If your partner is willing to provide this for you then they are a loving and caring partner because in the grand scheme of all this, headscissors truly aren't the craziest sexual desire to have. The higher degrees get dangerous, but compared to sounding, piss drinking, and castration stuff, this is light work. The bottom line is, if they hate it yet they do it for you…that says a lot about their love for you. Expectedly, you need to reward them! If someone does something for you, despite absolutely hating it, there is no other option but to show your appreciation for them. You know what the best act of appreciation is for your partner. It may be sexual, it may not. Do it, then do it again, and then do it a third time so they know you are serious. Make them feel appreciated.

After all of this, if they still say no to headscissoring you, refusing to settle for even the third or second degree, you have a choice to make...a lesson to learn. At this point, you will have to decide: *Is headscissoring my sexual desire...or is it my sexual need?* This will lead to a series of decisions.

First, ask your partner if they are okay with you fulfilling this need via session girls. If they say no, move on to the next paragraph. If they say yes, you get headscissored by session girls and have a loving girlfriend back home. Congratulations! While the headscissors may be empty in terms of fulfillment, the rest of your sexual fulfillment is waiting back at home with open and loving arms.

So your partner said no to headscissoring you and said absolutely not to you getting a paid headscissor session. You have two options:

**A.** Sacrifice your sexual desires for the relationship.
**B.** Sacrifice the relationship for your sexual needs.

Both of these outcomes are equally ***OKAY***. Never should you feel shame or guilt for sacrificing the relationship for your true sexual needs, and never should you harbor resentment for your partner for not agreeing to headscissor you. If you can't imagine spending the rest of your life with someone who refuses to keep you close in a reverse headscissor then pick option B. Your soul will thank you for putting yourself first, and you can spend your newly acquired free time searching for a partner who is willing to headscissor you.

However, if your partner is perfect in every single conceivable way with the exception of headscissoring, it is equally acceptable to say goodbye to all of your headscissor fantasies. There may be plenty of things you dislike about your partner, but if they refuse to headscissor you that doesn't automatically mean you have to leave them. At the end of the day, no matter how stressed you may be about your partner refusing to headscissor you or their opinion on headscissoring, it all comes down to you. Yay! More stress on your shoulders! I'm joking, but it is important to know that they are not required to fulfill this for you. If she refuses to fulfill your sexual desires YOU must decide if she is the partner for you, not her. It is best to know the answer to the following question before even communicating your potential sexual needs or desires to your partner. Is headscissoring a 'dealbreaker' for you? If so, to be headscissored is a sexual **NEED**. If not, it is a sexual **desire**. Both are perfect. Figure out if headscissoring is your need or desire before referring back to options **A** and **B**, and you will already know what to do in the case she isn't willing to try headscissoring.

"This is all too much. I just want to be scissored into bliss."

I can try to help. If talking about this with your partner is too nerve racking, stressful, or even inconvenient, I will happily help. Want to make a fun game out of it to cut some of the tension? I can help. What I need you to do is simple but tedious. For example, the next time you are with your partner on the couch, and things start getting spicy, stop. Say, "Wait. I need to talk to you about something." Retrieve this book and flip open to the 'dear beloved' page that will follow these paragraphs. Present the page to your partner after previously writing their name on the line. Then without saying a word leave the room. Ideally, go to a bedroom or another vacant room and wait patiently on the bed. If there is no bedroom, find somewhere…find anywhere in another room to wait patiently. No phone. No distractions. Just you. Once in a separate room, lay down on your back with your feet facing away from the door you entered through. Stare at the ceiling and wait. Not a single word should be uttered from your mouth while waiting. Eventually, your partner will wander into the room after you. Here she will either scoop you up in a reverse headscissor or tell you, "No." No meaning, she will never headscissor you.

By now you should already know what your response will be, whether you sacrifice your desires or sacrifice the relationship…you know. Will it be awkward to stand up and abandon the relationship, absolutely. At least you did it with dignity and on your terms though! If she does decide to scoop you up in a reverse please note, upon the first instant you feel dizzy or in too much pain, you must tap out. I will have communicated this with her, and she has been assured she won't hurt you badly or knock you unconscious. While you know headscissors are inherently uncomfortable to an extent, you must tap long before falling asleep every single time. I wish you the best of luck! I will also try my best to make the following gender neutral for anyone else wanting to convince their partner to headscissor them. Regardless, I advise you to read through it before deciding to present it to them.

# Dear Beloved

_____,

We need to talk about something important. Your partner has retreated to another room for a deeply significant reason. Please, don't rush after them just yet. They've asked you to read this alone first, as they're feeling incredibly nervous. To say they're anxious would be an understatement. Your loving partner is about to share something with you—a desire that many might have criticized, mocked, or even shunned them for. Is it sexual? Yes. Is it considered a little frisky? Perhaps. Will it bring them closer to you? Absolutely. Will you do it? That's the very question they're anxiously pondering.

I won't beat around the bush because time is of the essence. Your devoted partner wants to surrender sexual control to you. But before you panic and close this book in protest, let me explain what they're asking for. They want you to give them a headscissor session. "What!?" Yes, I'm relaying this on their behalf. While I, the author, am completely safe and unaffected where I wrote this, they are feeling vulnerable to your response. Oh... you meant... what as in... what is a headscissor? Well… in that case, what they want you to do is walk into the room after them, lay on their stomach facing their feet, and scoop their head up between your thighs. That is pretty much it. No, it isn't anything too extreme. Not much different from oral, which is, pardon my candor, something I encouraged them to enthusiastically provide you already. If this feels too overwhelming, it's okay to close the book and kindly decline. Don't say anything else. Just go to them and say no. While it might disappoint them, at least they'll have a clear answer. They will understand this will never be an option in the relationship, and if they are accepting of that you both can continue your journey together.

If, however, you're happy or willing to provide this gesture for your partner regularly, then I'll guide you through making it the highlight of their week, if not their month or even year. Are you ready? Start by setting a timer on your phone for anywhere between ten and twenty minutes. When the timer goes off, the headscissoring ends. "But what if I hurt them?" That's a valid concern. Rest assured, they're aware of what's happening. While it may not seem like it, they've likely considered this scenario before, and chances are, they've even read over these exact pages explaining what you're about to do. Set the timer.

Now, when you walk into that room… don't say a word. Get down on your knees, and make sure that your knees are touching each side of your partner's head. Lean forward so that the rest of your body is being supported by your hands like those half push-ups we all did in elementary. Then drop your groin down to their upper chest or collar bone. Make sure their head is nicely placed between your legs, their ears should be in the middle of your thighs. Then wiggle backwards to press your butt into their face. While doing this use one of your calves to lift their head off the ground and push it further between your cheeks. You can use your hands to help pull their face in closer if you need to. Once you get them in there nice and deep, stretch out the leg you used to lift their head and cross your ankles.

They should, in theory, just barely be able to see over your butt, but this can change depending on your size and their size. Don't squeeze at all and don't stretch much at all either, just hold them there. Lastly, wrap your arms around their body and hug them. Lay your head to rest on their body and simply hug them.

Euphoria. Utter euphoria. That is what they are feeling after you do that. Obviously, ten or so minutes of this will be boring. After a couple minutes they might want you to start squeezing, jiggling, or stretching harder. Whenever you are ready, do just that. My best advice is to slowly stretch out your legs until they are completely stretched. If at any point your partner repeatedly taps you, return to the hug position or release them completely. *That is the safe word, and they understand this too.* Anyways, stretch or squeeze slightly harder until they can't handle the hold. Never squeeze as hard as you can. Take this time to get to better understand your own strength in a way you probably never have before. Your partner wants this for you, and is willing to help you learn more about yourself. They want you to feel powerful. They want to bask in the glory of your inescapable strength, just like you would want to bask in theirs.

Once again, make sure their head is positioned so that your thighs are squeezing their ears like earmuffs. Of course, you can position your thighs around their neck if you so choose, but just be extra careful and sensitive to your partner's reaction once you start stretching because you could unintentionally choke them. Regardless, they will love the view, and this will allow you to practice your jiggle game and glute squeeze if you so choose. With that being said, don't get overwhelmed. It may seem like a lot to do, but I will sum it up one last time for you. Then I will provide some example photos to help you visualize the near future. I wish you the best of luck!

Timer? SET.

Partner? FOUND.

Their head? KNEES PARALLEL.

Their waist? LEANED FORWARD ABOVE.

Your crotch? RESTING ON THEIR UPPER CHEST.

Their head? BETWEEN YOUR LEGS.

Your buttcheeks? SLIGHTLY SPREAD BY THEIR NOSE.

Your calf and heel? LIFTING THEIR HEAD INTO POSITION.

Your legs and ankles? SOFTLY LOCKING THEM IN POSITION.

You? HUGGING YOUR PARTNER'S LOWER HALF.

Everybody? EUPHORIC AND ENJOYING THE INTIMACY.

What now? YOU PLAY AROUND WITH THEM LIKE A SHOW OFF.

First photo, example of step 3: Knees parallel.

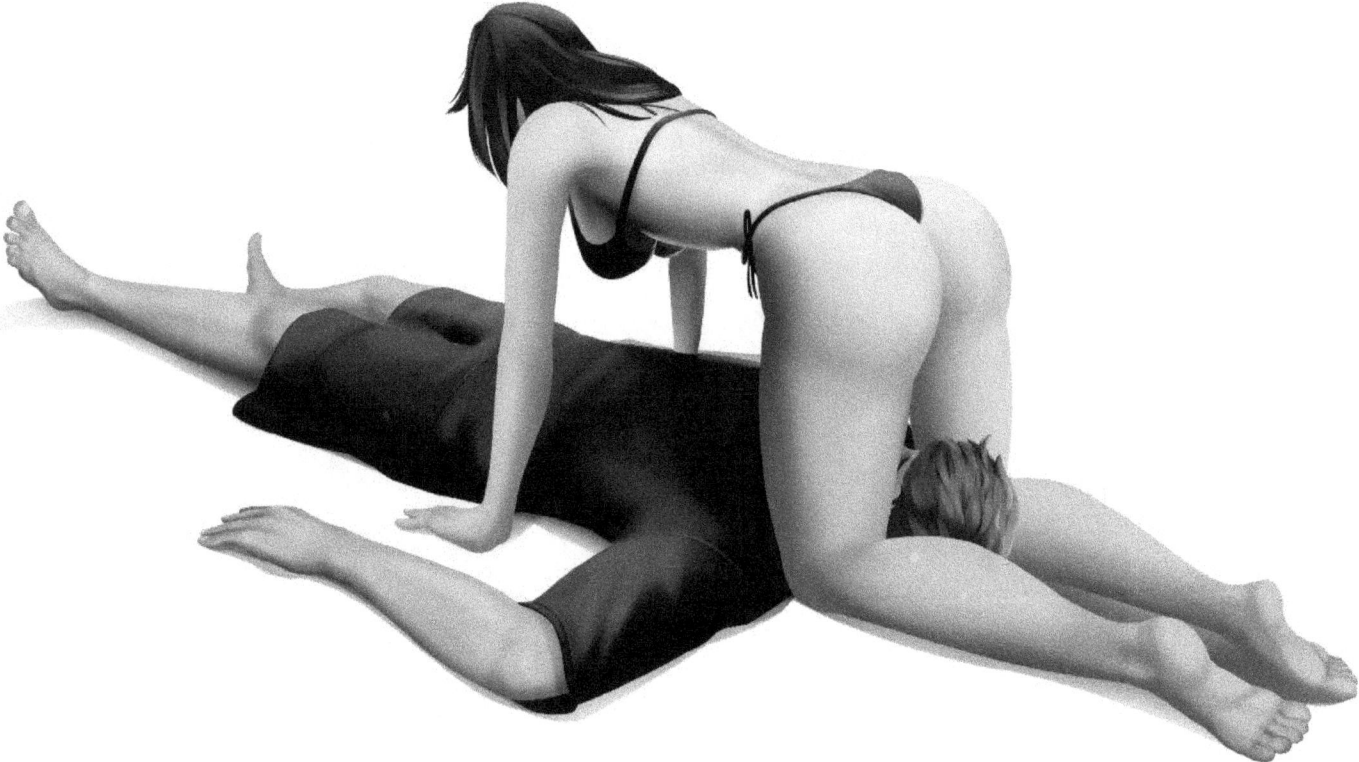

Second photo, example of step 4 and 5: Leaned forward and crotch/waist above chest.

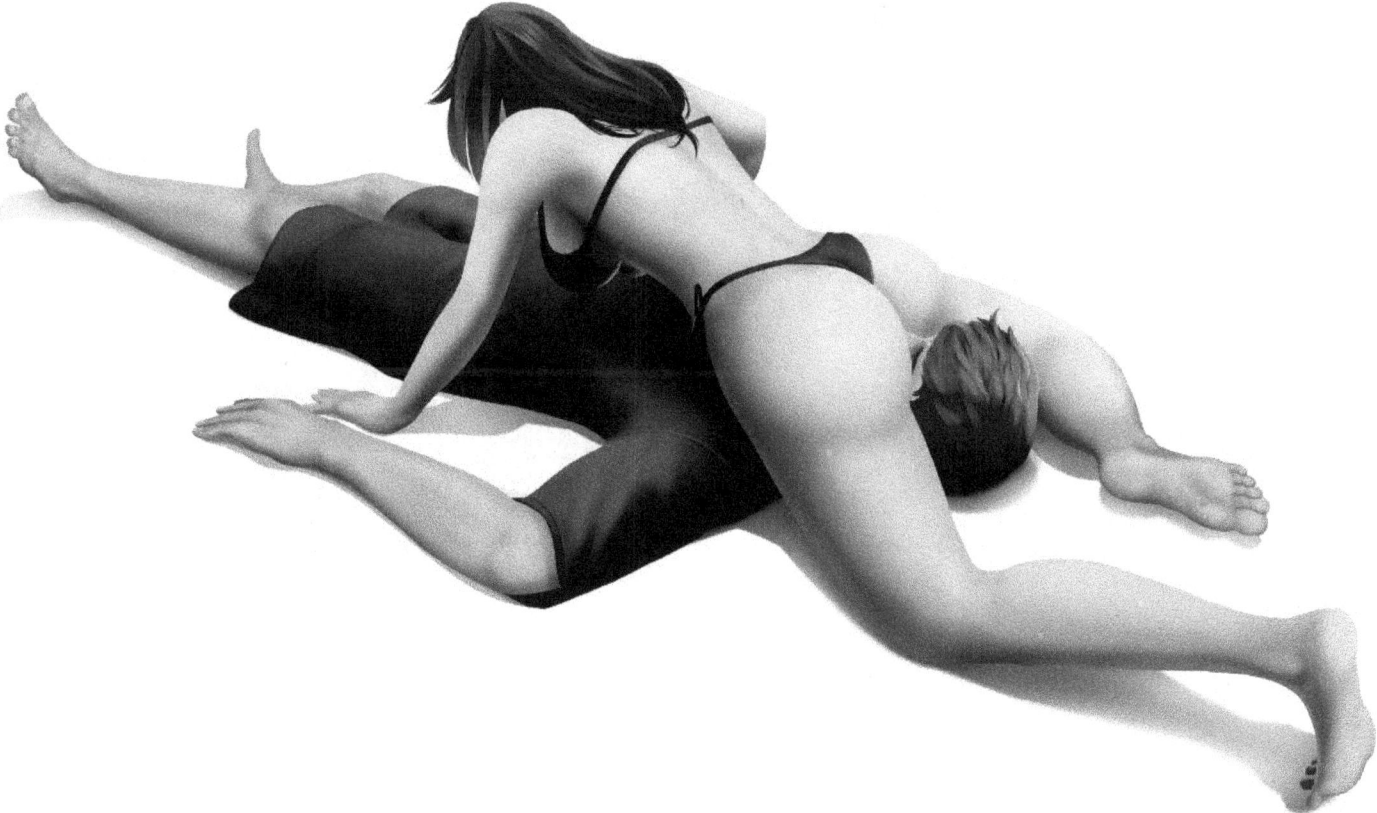

Third photo, example of step 7 and 8: Using your calf or ankle to lift their head off the floor and deeper into your butt.

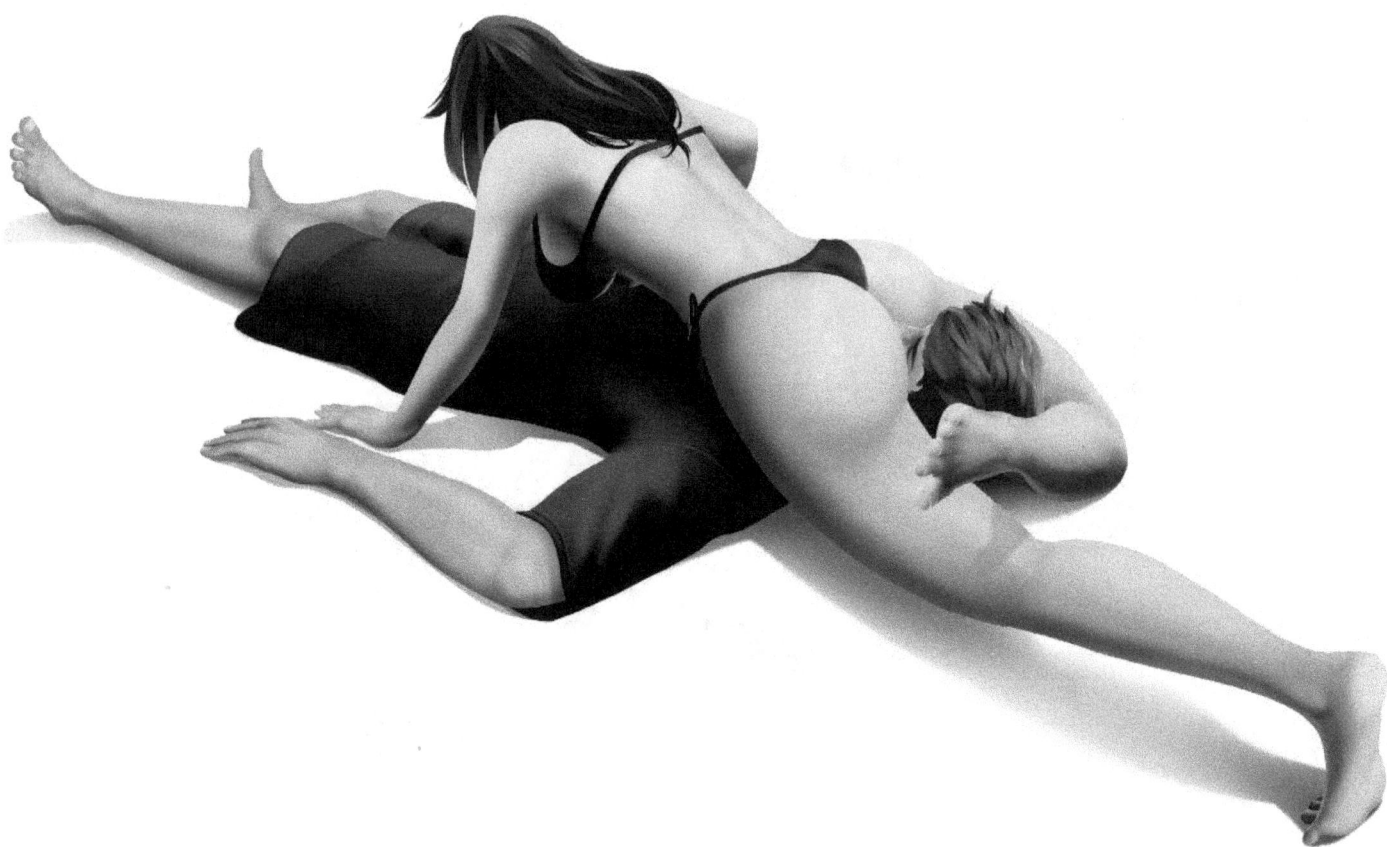

Fourth photo, example of step 9: Locking them in place by stretching legs and crossing ankles.

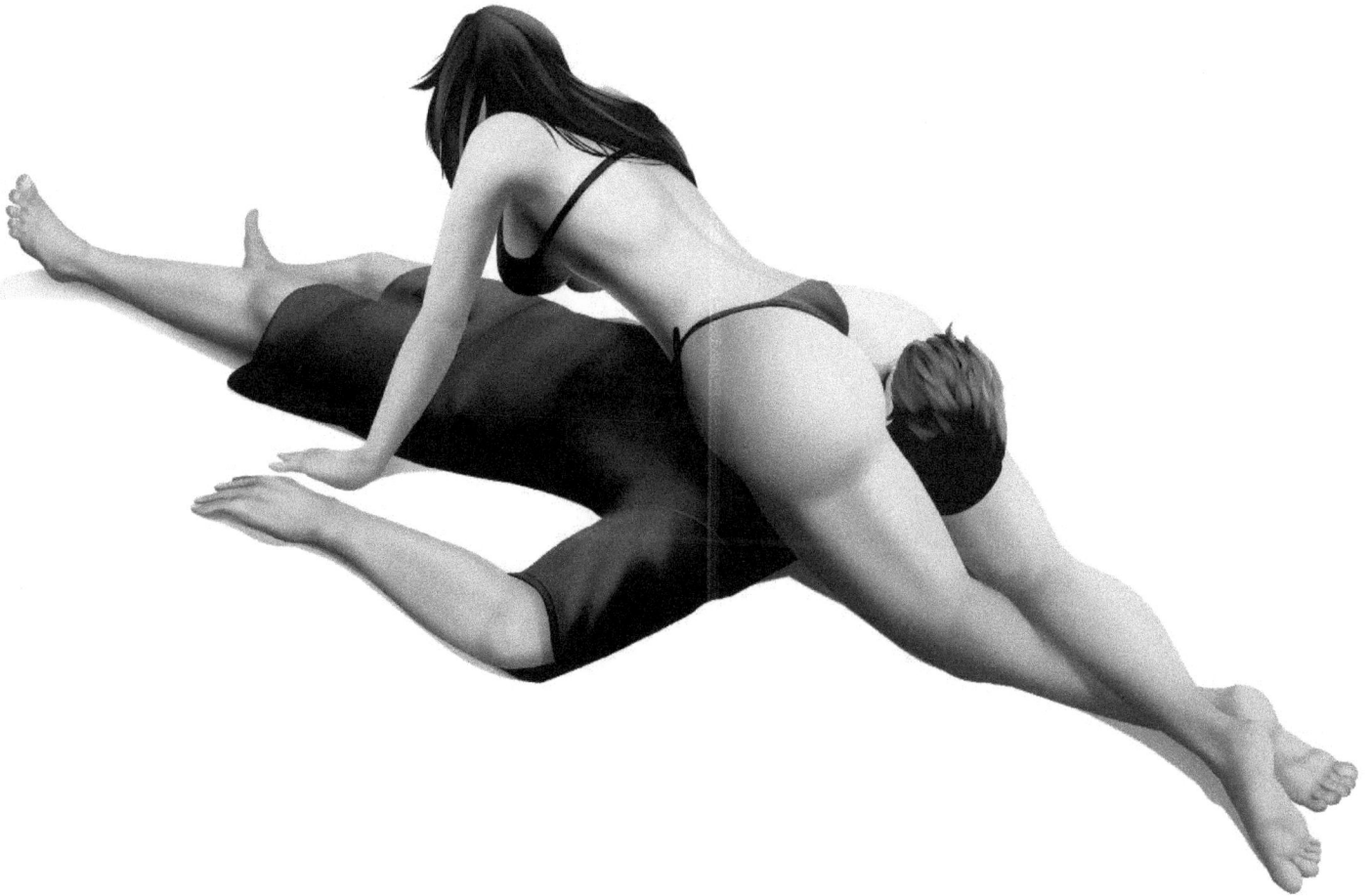

# Chapter 6

## Types of Headscissors

Ah, yes. The plentiful types of headscissoring. Easily one of the more interesting chapters. Here we will learn about all the different positions, holds, and miscellaneous headscissor facts that can increase your headscissor skills. It is important to note that the naming of these headscissor was done by me, the author. In the real world (not sexual) such as martial arts or wrestling the name of one position can vary and certain wrestlers may make their own names for positions and so forth. I tried to follow the general consensus on naming, but I added some directionally assisting aspects to the name process. For example, if it is *Front* that means the person applying the hold is looking at their victim. *Feet Facing* means that the victim is looking away or towards the feet of the person applying the headscissors. *Reverse* means the person applying the scissor is looking away from their victim and so forth. With that note existing for you to digest, let us get straight into it with the different types and positions.

**Front Headscissor/Standard Headscissor**. Also known as just a headscissor, the front facing headscissor is the standard in the field. The main thing to notice here is that the female gets to watch her victim directly. It can be done in a variety of ways, but we will focus only on two of them. The male's head is gripped between the thighs which stretch outwards and lock at the ankles. The female can be laying on her back looking directly into the eyes of her victim, or she can be sitting on his chest where his head, facing her, is scooped between her thighs. Her legs can stretch out straight behind his head or extend out at multiple different angles. This is the best position to attempt your first knockout regardless of gender, as the one in control will witness the victim slip away without having to turn, bend, or stretch around themself.

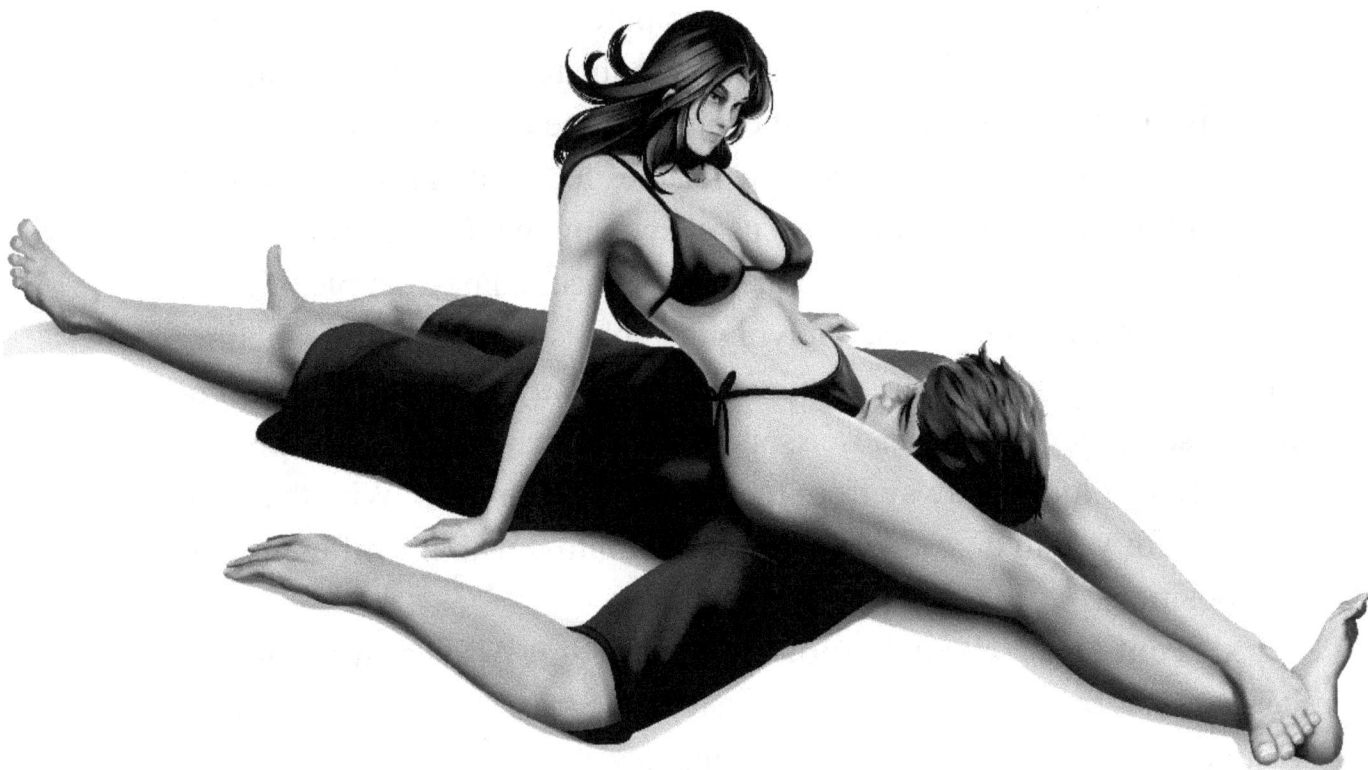

**Front Headscissor on Side**. This is the exact same as the previous with the exception that both parties are laying down on their sides. The female uses her hips to flip him completely onto his side which increases pressure. This position adds additional pressure to the male as her leg is being pulled down on his neck by gravity. To reduce this pain one can rest his head on a pillow so that gravity doesn't pull the full weight of his head into her other leg. Pain, however, is guaranteed in this position.

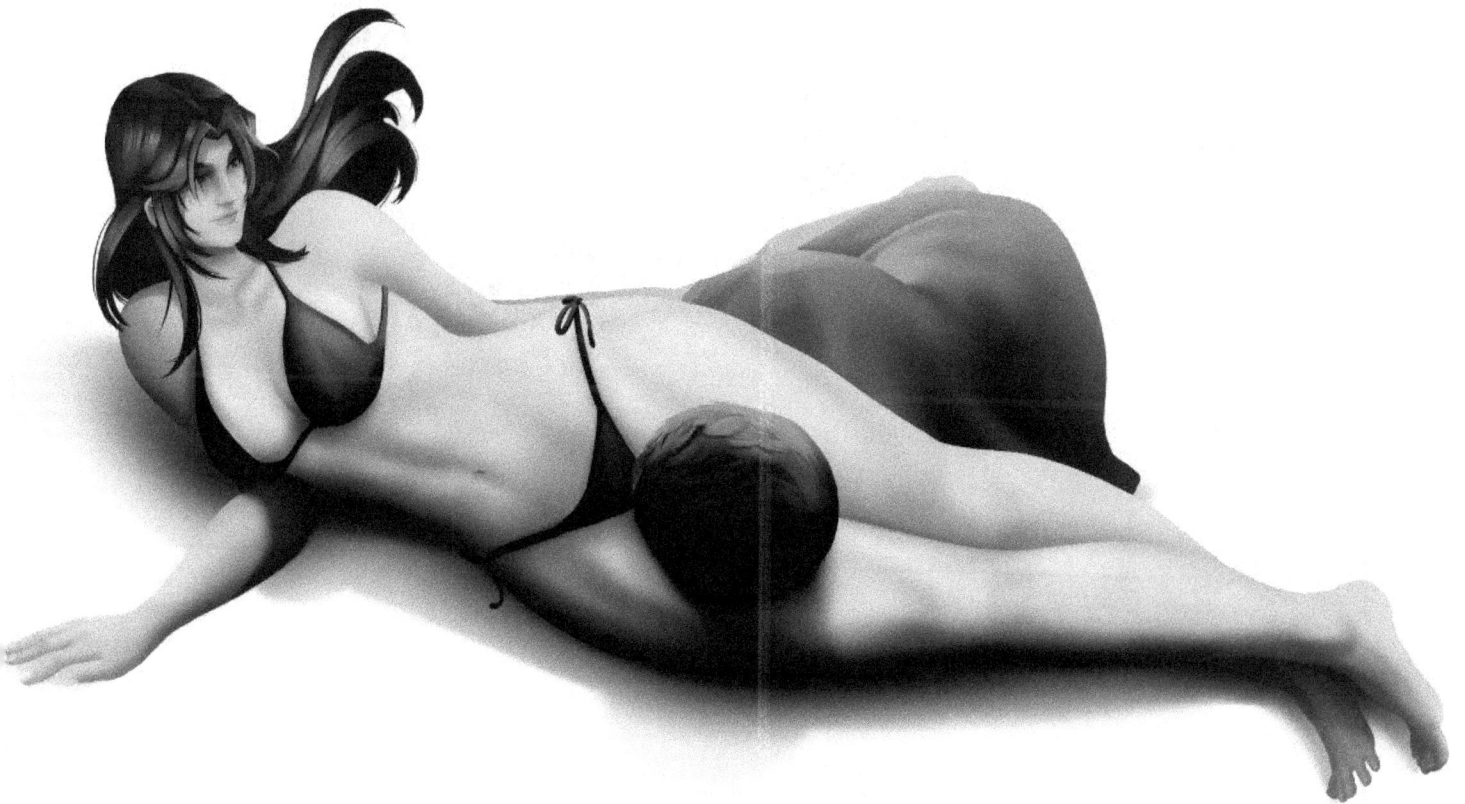

**Feet Facing Headscissor**. A variation similar to the front headscissor is the feet facing headscissor. As one could guess, he is facing her feet, and she gets to watch the back of his head. This can also be done in many variations: laying, standing, kneeling, on the side, etc.

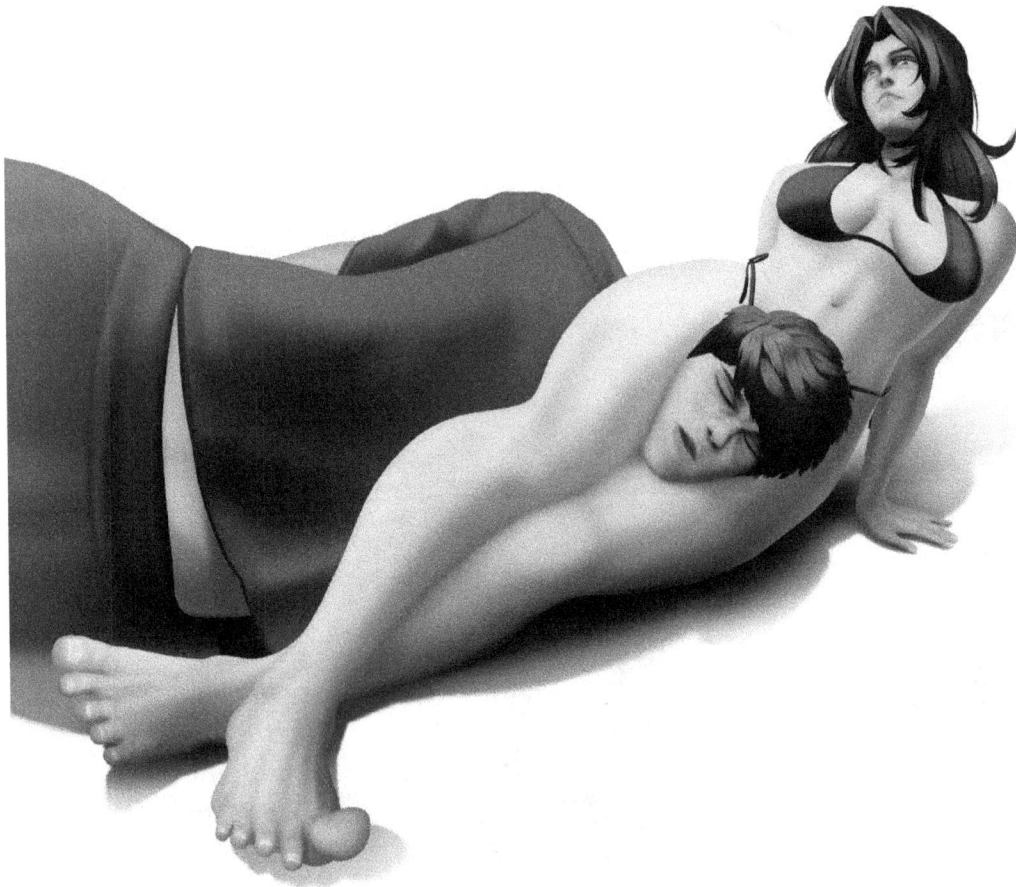

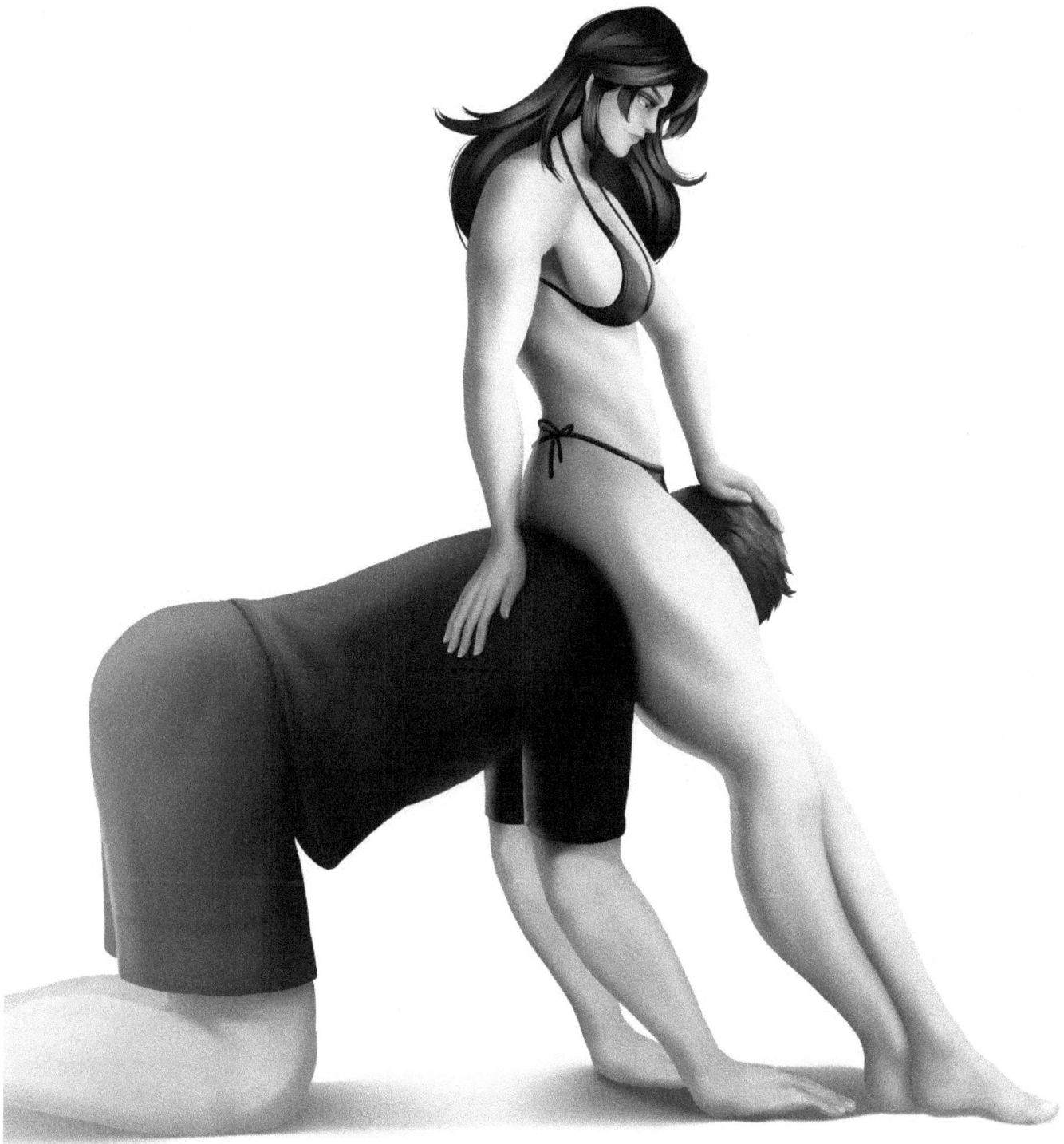

**Side Headscissor**. A side headscissor is a move where the female applying the hold is positioned at the side of the male, using her legs to scissor the man's head or neck from the front and back rather than the sides. This can be extremely painful and dangerous since the trachea experiences much more pressure. I advise to never attempt this type of headscissor at all due to the pure risk the placement provides. The main difference between this and the front headscissor on side is that he is laying on his back looking up, and the female is laying on her side facing either way.

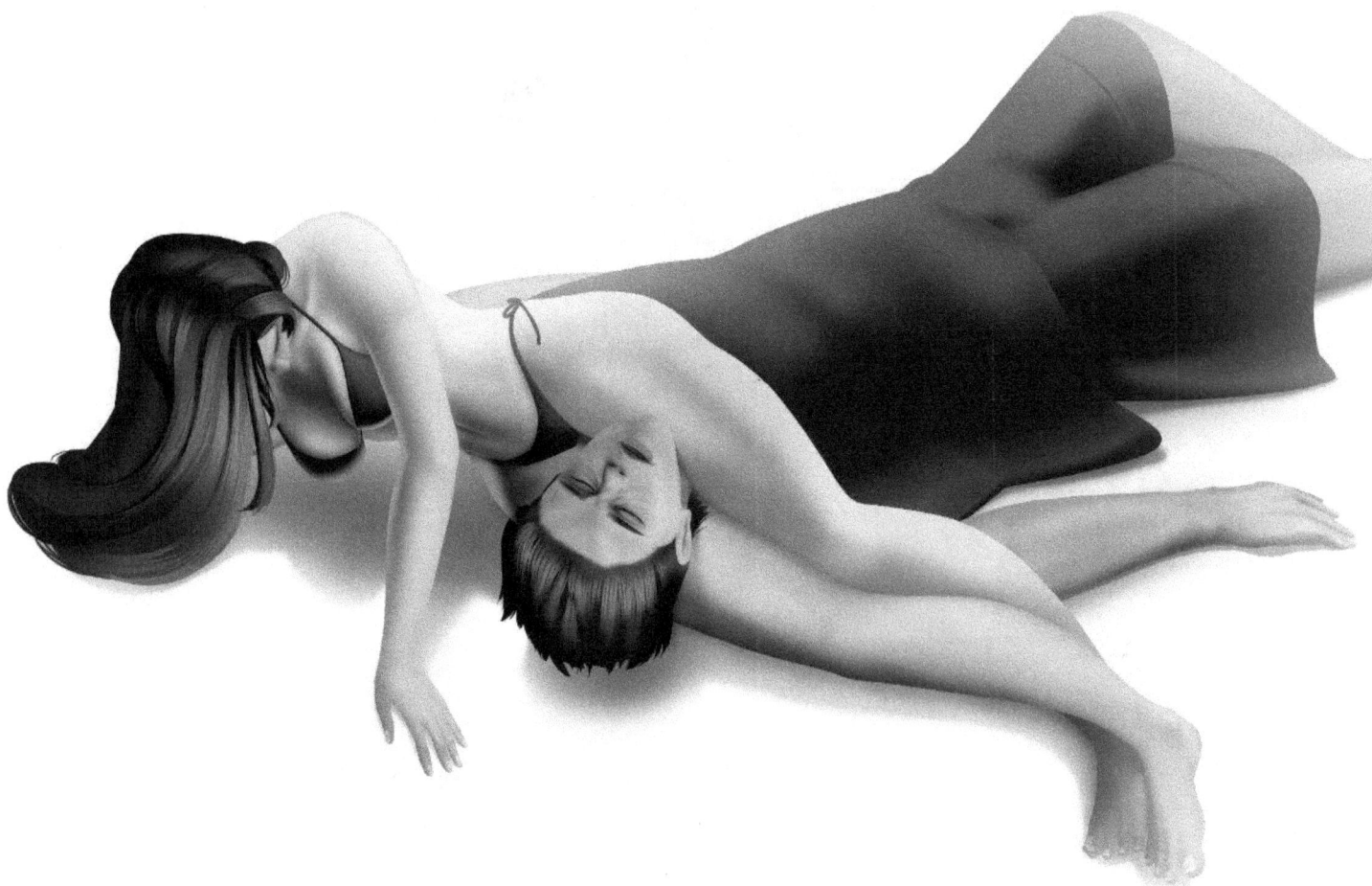

**Reverse Headscissor**. The reverse and all of its variations has the female facing away from her victim. It is easily one of the most popular positions and for great reason. In a standard reverse headscissor, the male lays flat on his back and the female scoops him up, stuffing his face or throat into her butt. This is one of the most powerful headscissors because it adds an additional muscle to the fight, the glutes. As crazy as it sounds, not only do the thighs squeeze the victim, but the glutes can also apply pressure leading to some of the fastest knockouts ever possible. For the men the view adds tremendously to the experience, and if you are a woman the absolute control you have in this position is unrivaled. The ease at which most of the woman's glutes can put him to sleep combined with the fact that his least futile attempt of escape is trying to pry apart her buttcheeks or thighs in feverish desperation makes this position so overpowered. In addition, the female has unrestricted access to the male's entire lower body. Once the legs are locked in place, she can pull him in as close as possible to her butt before she squeezes her thighs and glutes in tandem to create overwhelming pressure on his neck, leading to a hasty submission everytime or serving as a nasty means of control over him.

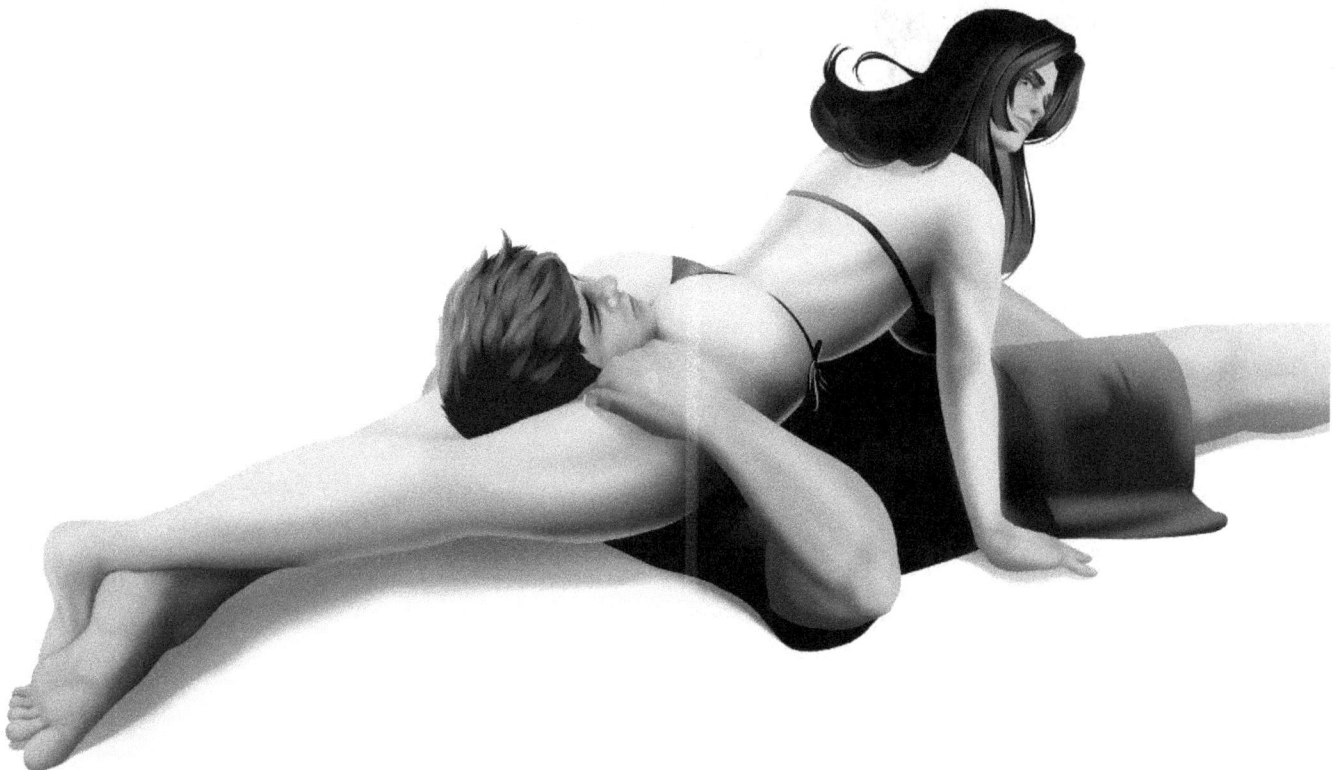

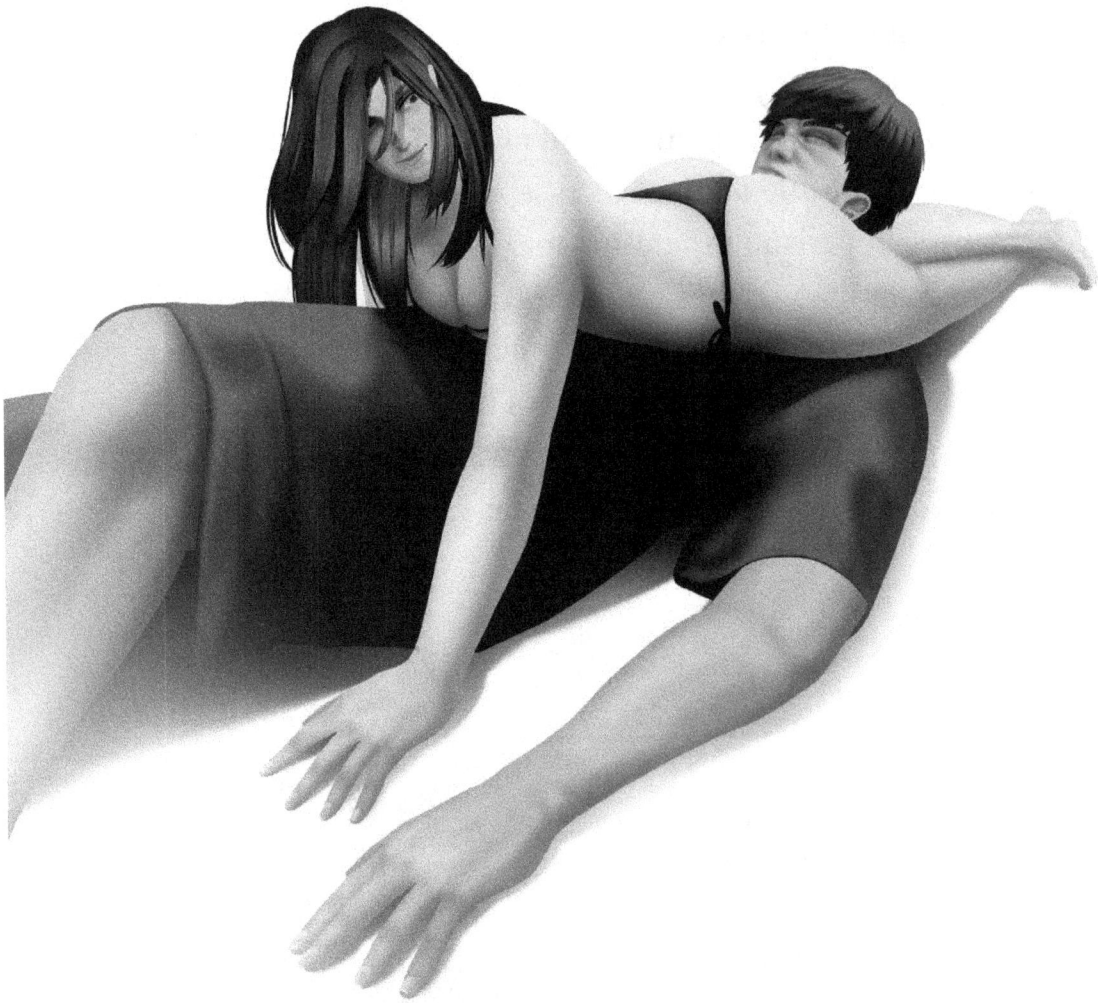

**Standing Reverse Headscissor**. This is the exact same as the previous, but instead of laying on the victim, the female stands adjacent to where the victim's head and neck hang off the side of whatever they are laying on. The female can still lean forwards or backwards at various angles, but the key concept is that the male's head is hanging off the edge of something which allows the woman to take a stand of a position of even more control.

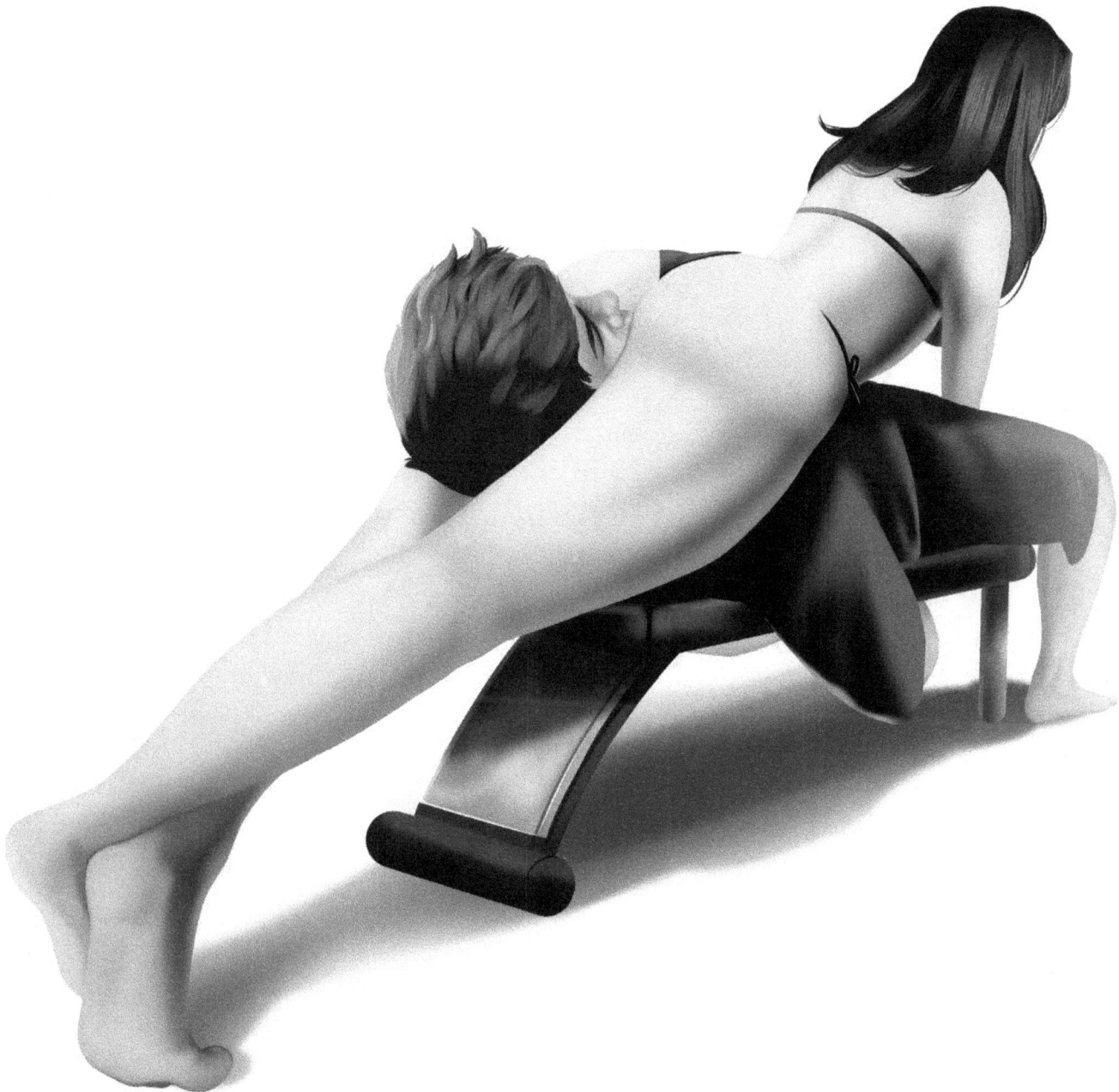

**Reverse Headscissor on Side**. The perfect combination of the reverse headscissor and the front headscissor on the side. Yet again the victim's face or head is scooped deep into the butt of the woman, but she rolls onto her side keeping him locked in tight. This can be in a sixty-nine position or a position where the male is perpendicular to the female. The added pressure from gravity ensures some pain, but the view is enough to keep most pleased in this position. Once again, pillows can help alleviate some pressure, if desired.

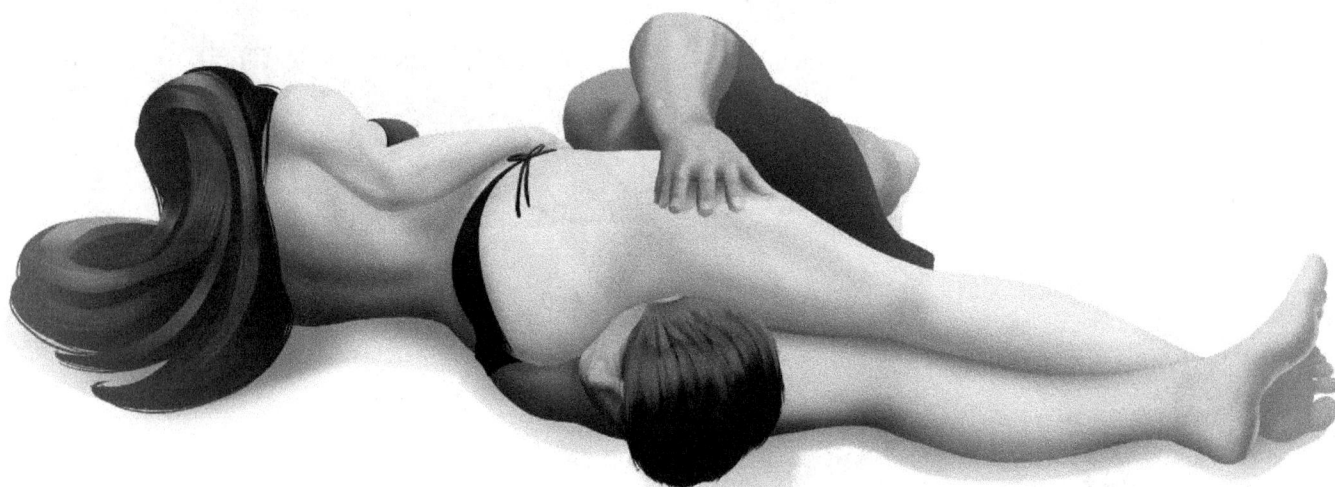

**Feet Facing Reverse Headscissor**. Think reverse headscissor. Now, imagine the male is facing away at the female's feet. Typically difficult to complete.

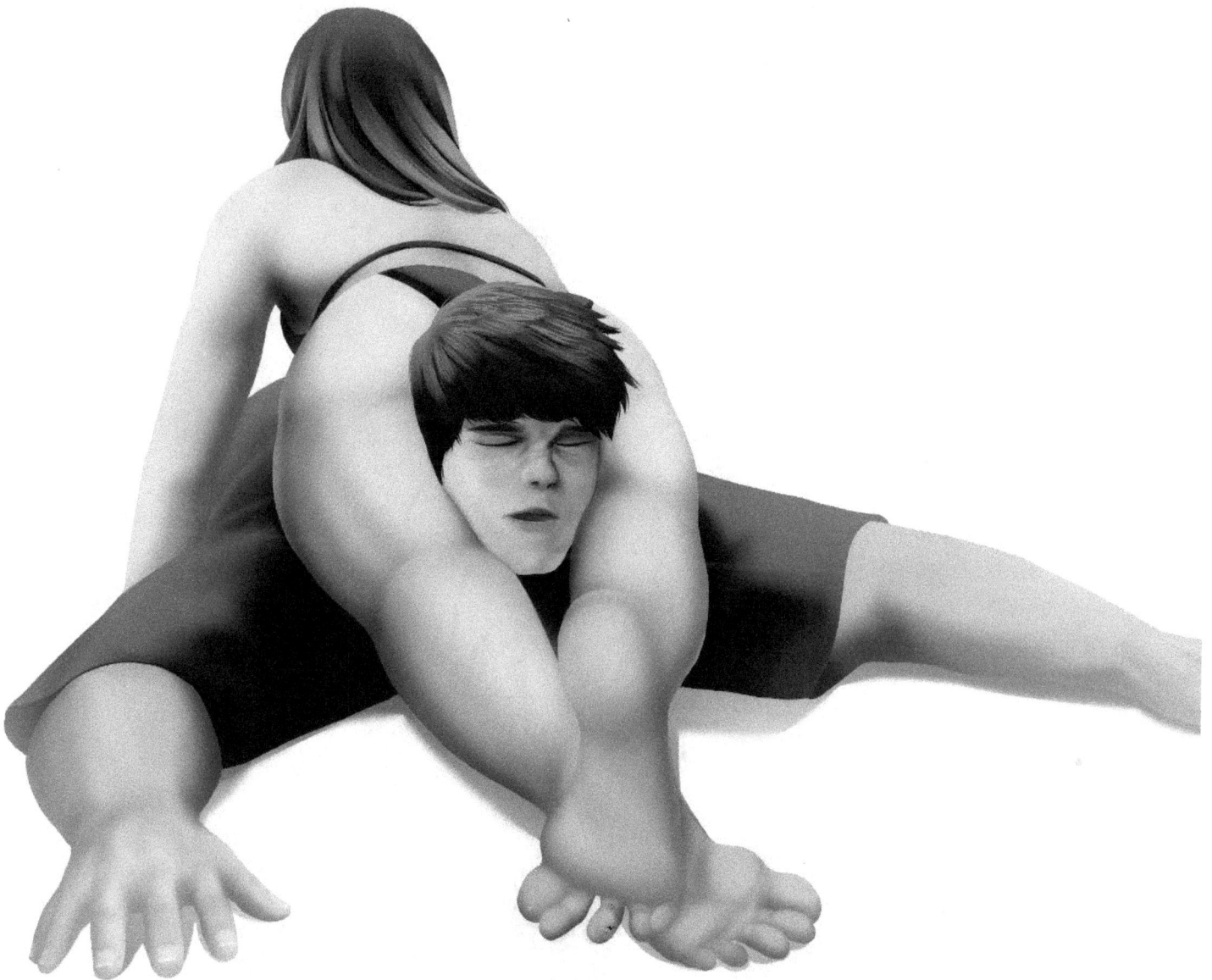

**Classic Hybrid**. This is the classic mix between the standard headscissor and a figure four. This can occur in all different variations, but typically only exists briefly before the legs lock out in a figure four or standard headscissor. The male's head is poking up between the female's thighs. It can face one of two ways: towards the female's head (Classic Hybrid and Reverse Hybrid) or over the knees to the female's feet (Feet Facing Hybrid and Reverse Feet Facing Hybrid). The female crosses her legs at the calf for this squeeze. If she were to stretch out completely it would turn into a standard headscissor, which one is based on where the male's head is facing. If she pulls one leg perpendicular to the other and locks it behind the calf of the extended leg it turns into a figure four.

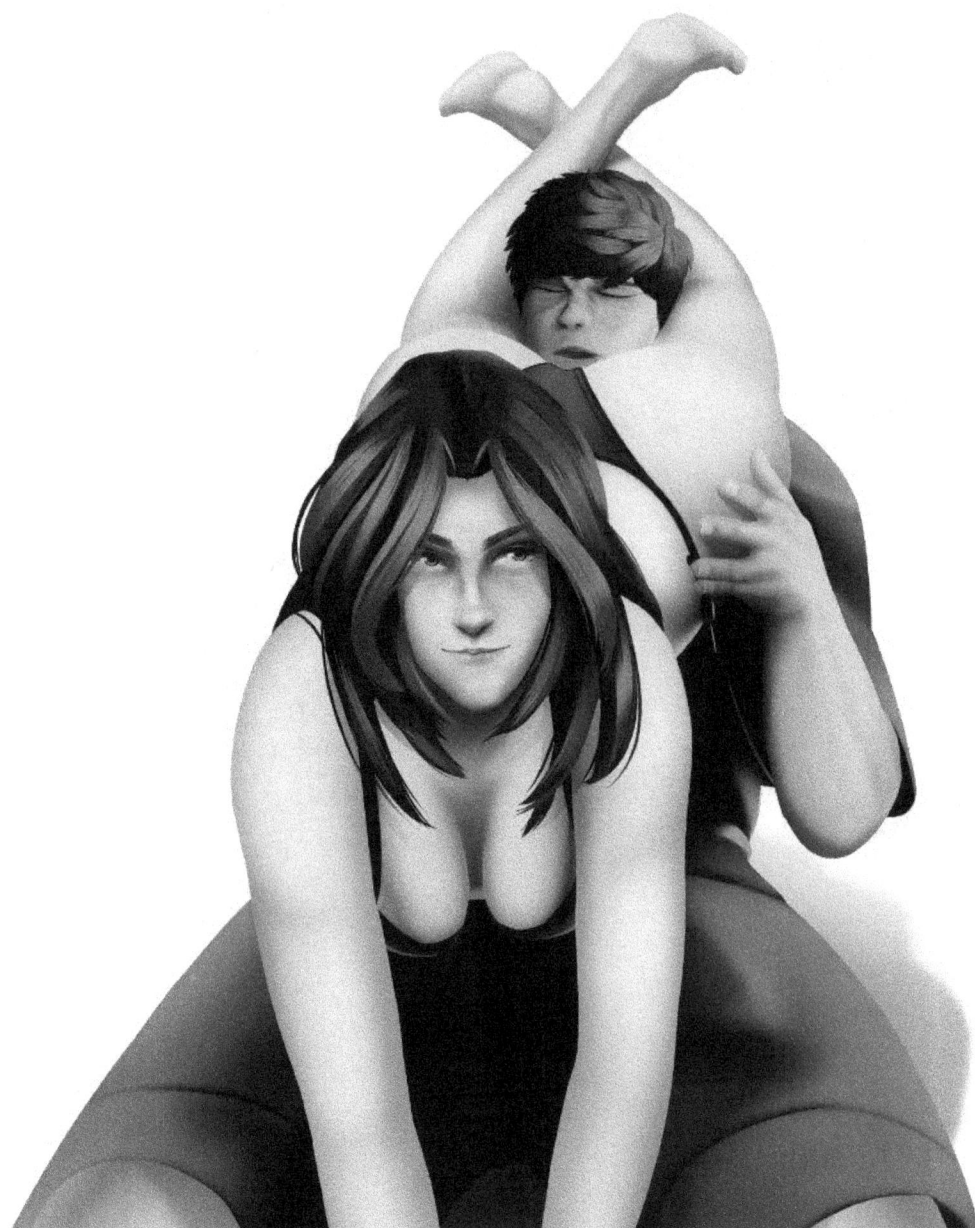

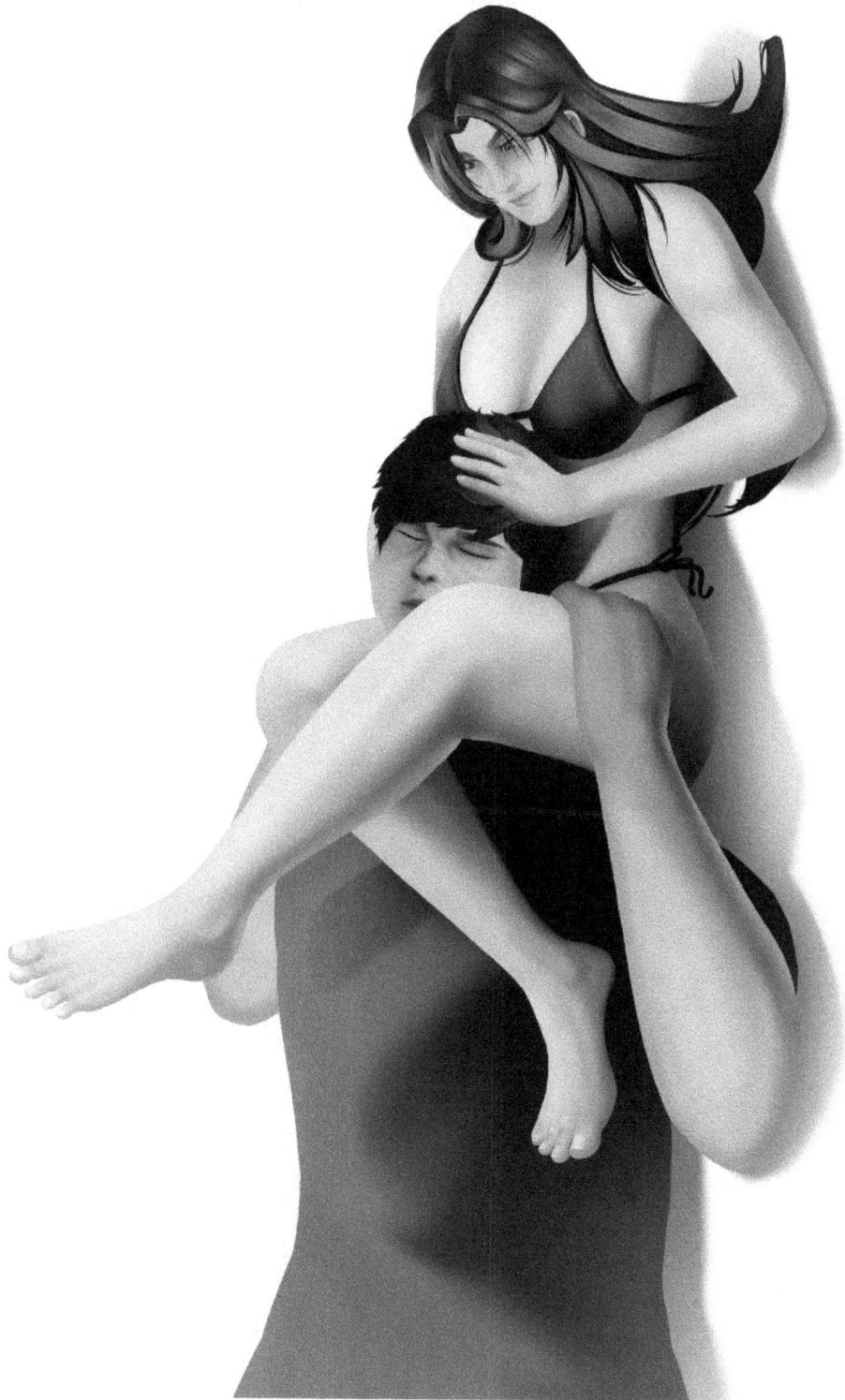

**Figure Four**. A standard Figure-Four Headscissor typically involves a woman using her legs to secure her man's head and neck in a manner that resembles the shape of the number "4." It also can be referred to as a triangle choke. It should be noted that in the headscissoring context figure fours are applied more so in a smothering manner. In the wrestling world however, a figure four focuses more on trapping the front of the victim's neck in the knee pit (behind the knee) where the carotid arteries can be squeezed by the calf and thigh for a quick and painless knockout. By no means does that mean you can't attempt the wrestling variant.

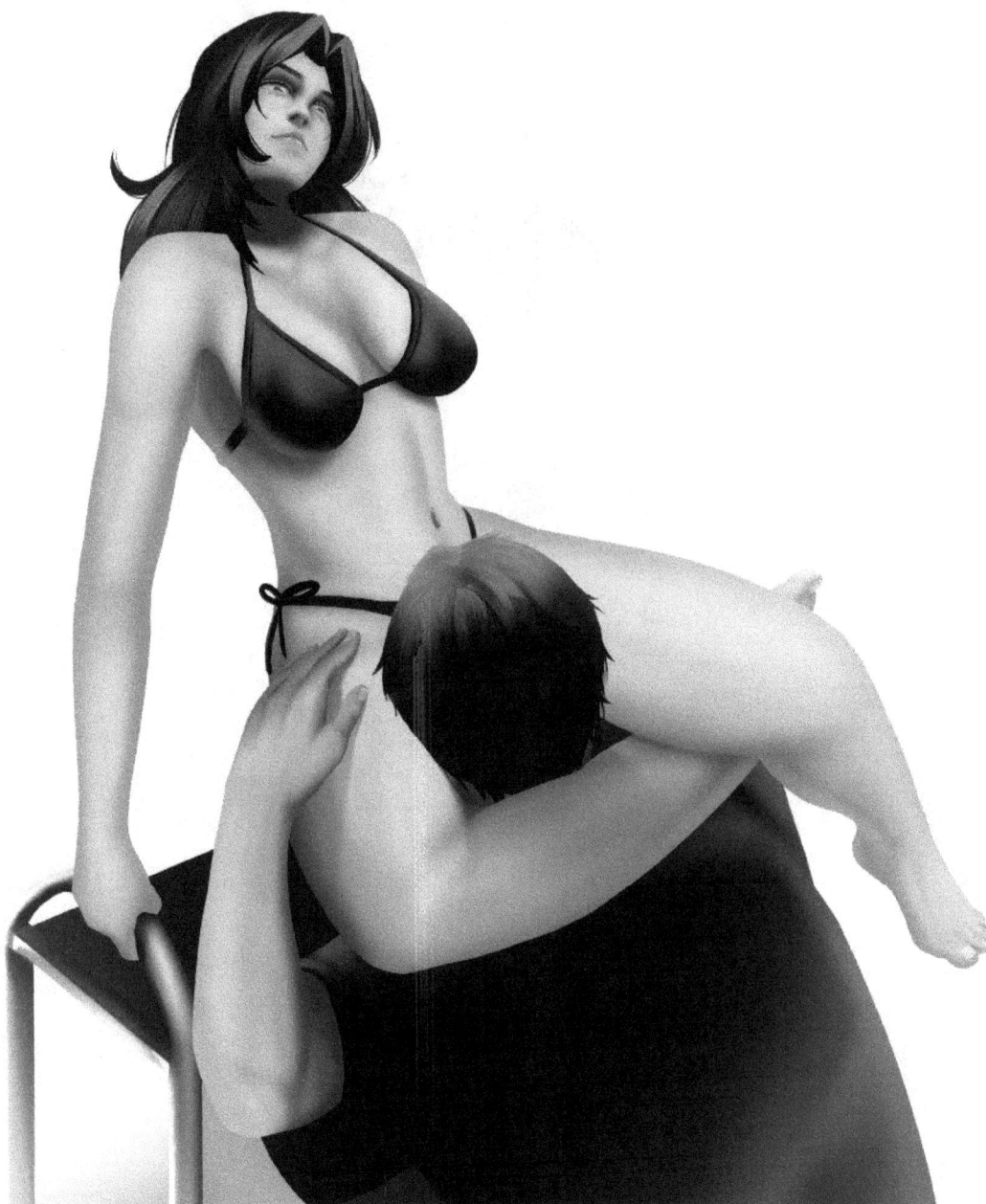

**Reverse Figure Four**. The perfect mix between the fabled reverse headscissor and the deadly figure four. Escape rates fall drastically from <1% to 0% when the woman grabs her foot to secure the victim in her grip.

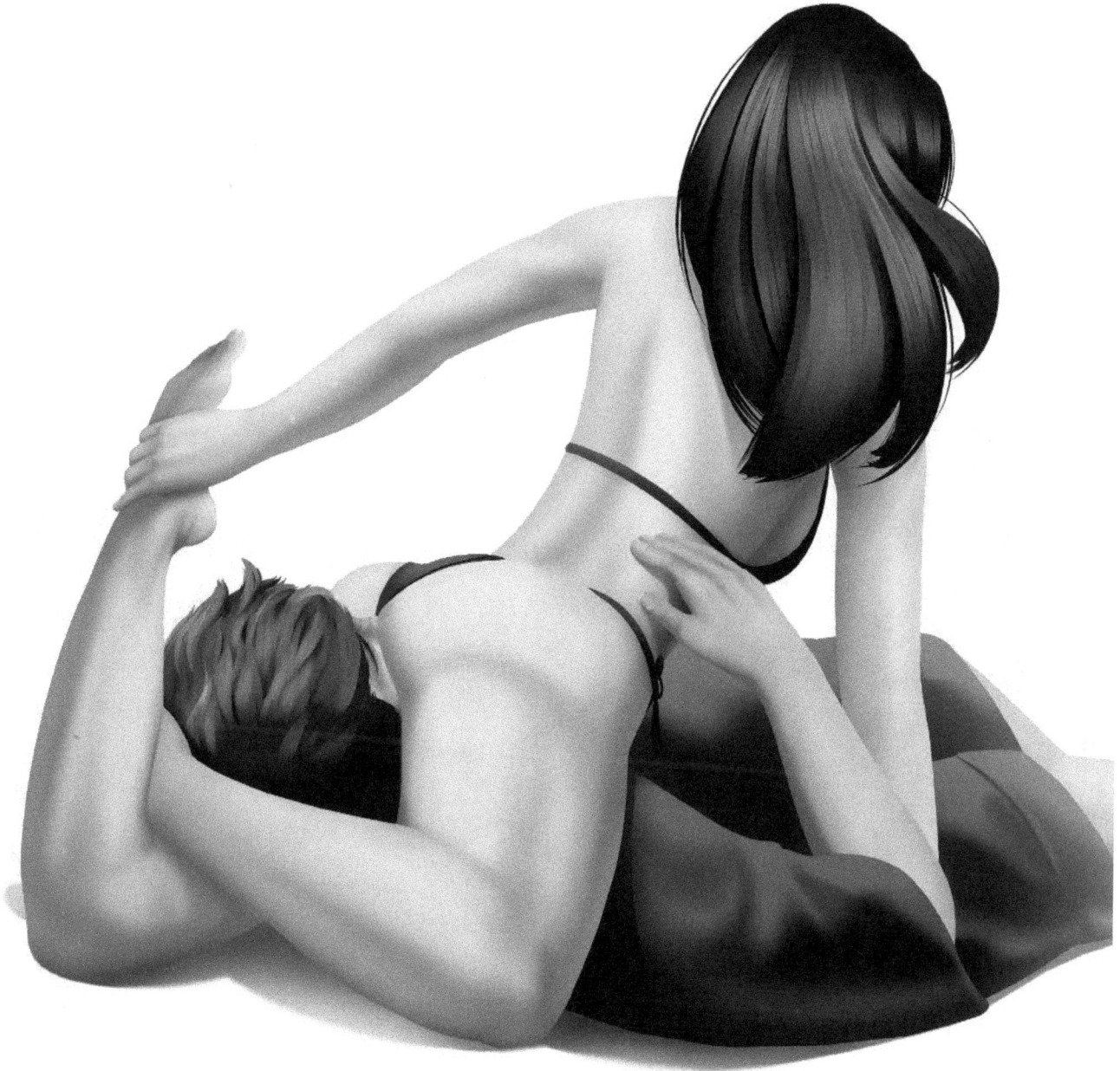

**Feet Facing Figure Four**. This is a figure four where the male faces away from the female, and it typically is more common and easier to complete than the other types of figure fours.

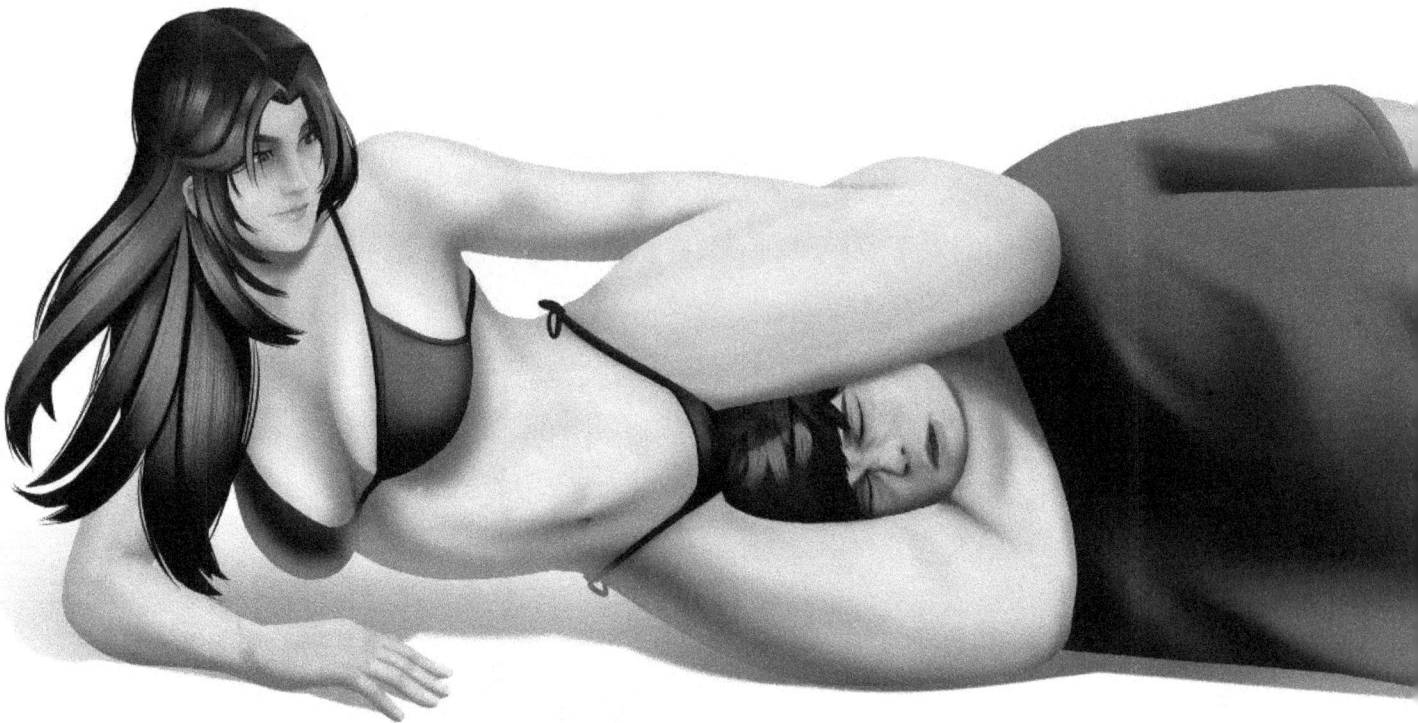

**Feet Facing Reverse Figure Four**. The most difficult to complete, both the male and the female are facing opposite directions. Think Feet facing reverse headscissor + figure four.

**Facesitting**. While not something you'd necessarily think of as headscissoring, facesitting technically can fall into the first and second degree of headscissoring if the head is straddled by the legs. If headscissoring is the valedictorian of their graduating high school class, then facesitting is the older sister that made the dean's list all through college and is also graduating as the valedictorian.

The acts are very similar so it would be wrong to leave facesitting out, but in preference of not getting too deep into it I will only hit the highlights since a whole book could be written on facesitting alone. Regardless, facesitting is where the woman sits on the man's face to create sexual pleasure for the both of them in a plethora of ways. It is really that simple. She can either be looking past the top of his head (Forward) or looking towards his feet (Reverse). In the **Forward Facesitting** position the male typically is closer to the female's vulva, and she is looking past his head. In the **Reverse Facesitting** position his face is closer to her butt, typically smothered completely under it, and she is facing his feet. Of course, just like headscissors, this can be done completely nude or completely clothed and standing or seated. We will talk a little bit more about facesitting in the next chapter.

Forward facesitting:

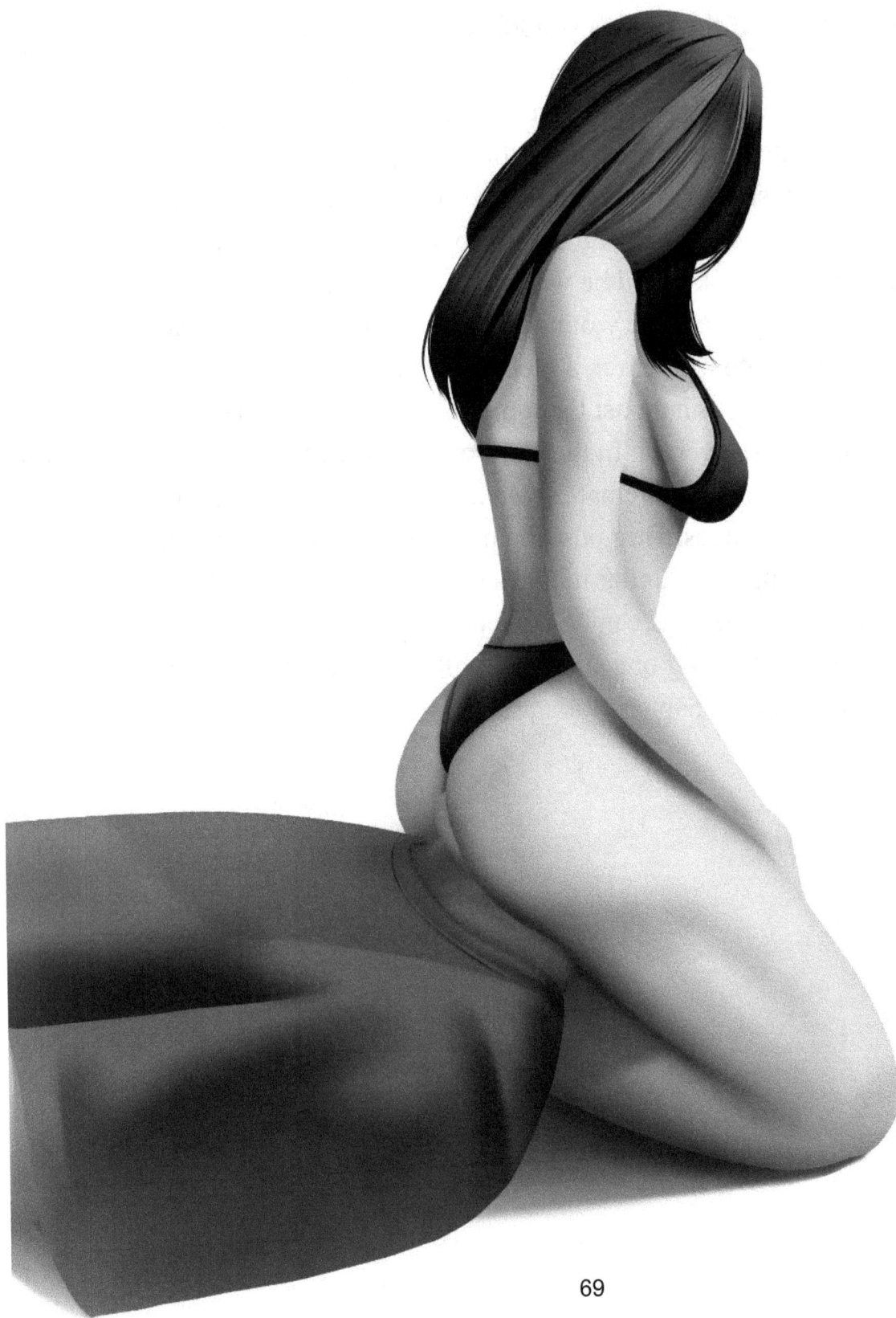

Reverse facesitting:

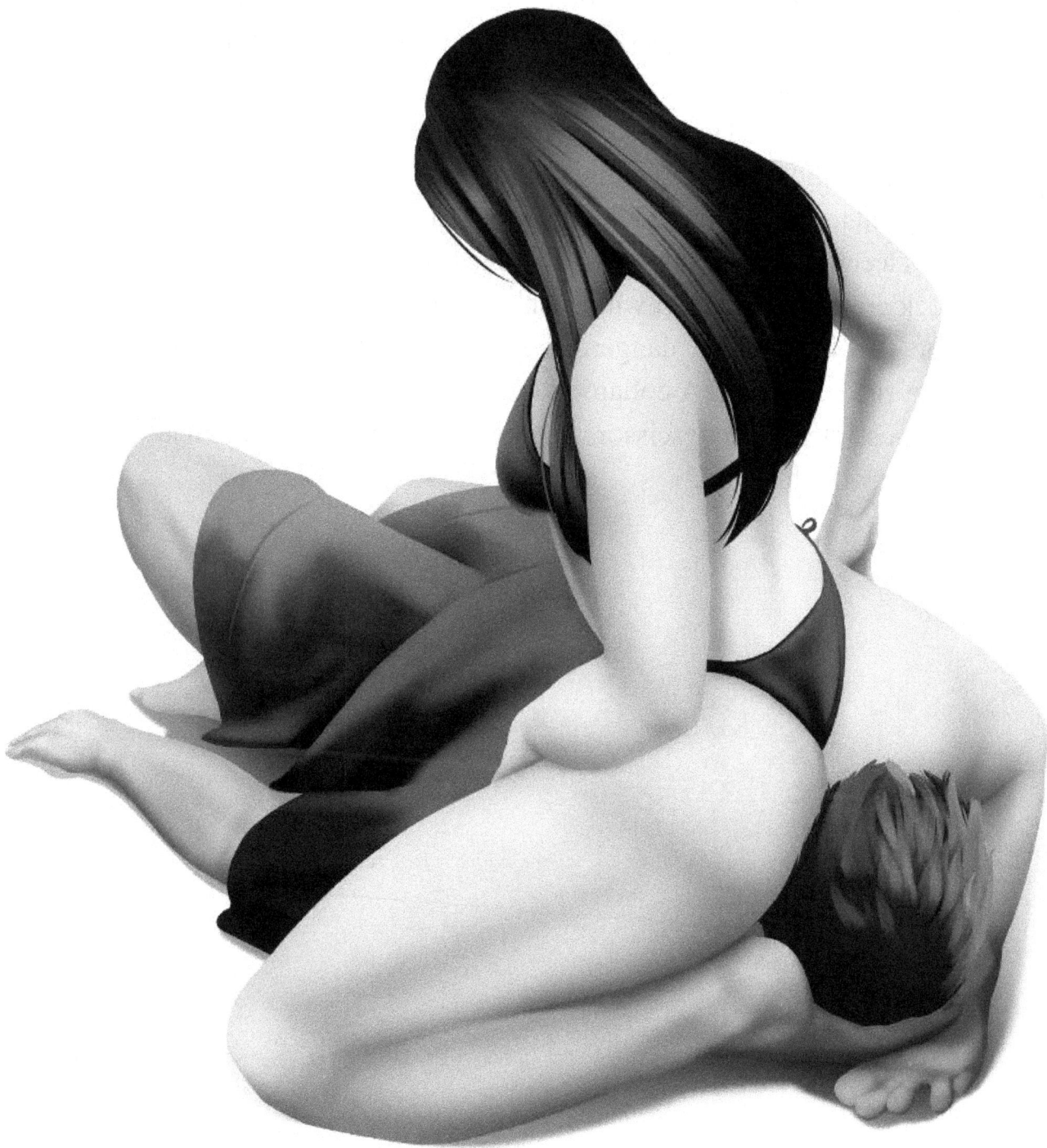

**Full-Weight Facesitting**. In this variation, the woman sits on the face of her man with her full body weight, providing a sense of extreme pressure and closeness.

**Teasing or Smothering Facesitting**. Some individuals may incorporate elements of teasing or smothering into facesitting, which can involve controlling the partner's access to breath for short periods or focusing on sensory play.

**Bodyscissors**. In a classic bodyscissors, the female wraps her legs around the male's midsection, creating a scissoring effect. The pressure is typically applied to the ribs or abdomen. I won't get too in depth with bodyscissors techniques, but as a guide if the legs can lock or even partially lock around a body part which isn't the head or neck, consider it a bodyscissor. This is extremely dangerous due to the fact that lots of vital organs are at risk of rupture. A collapsed lung, broken ribs, or other related risks are all possible in a bodyscissor, so take EXTREME caution when experimenting with this hold.

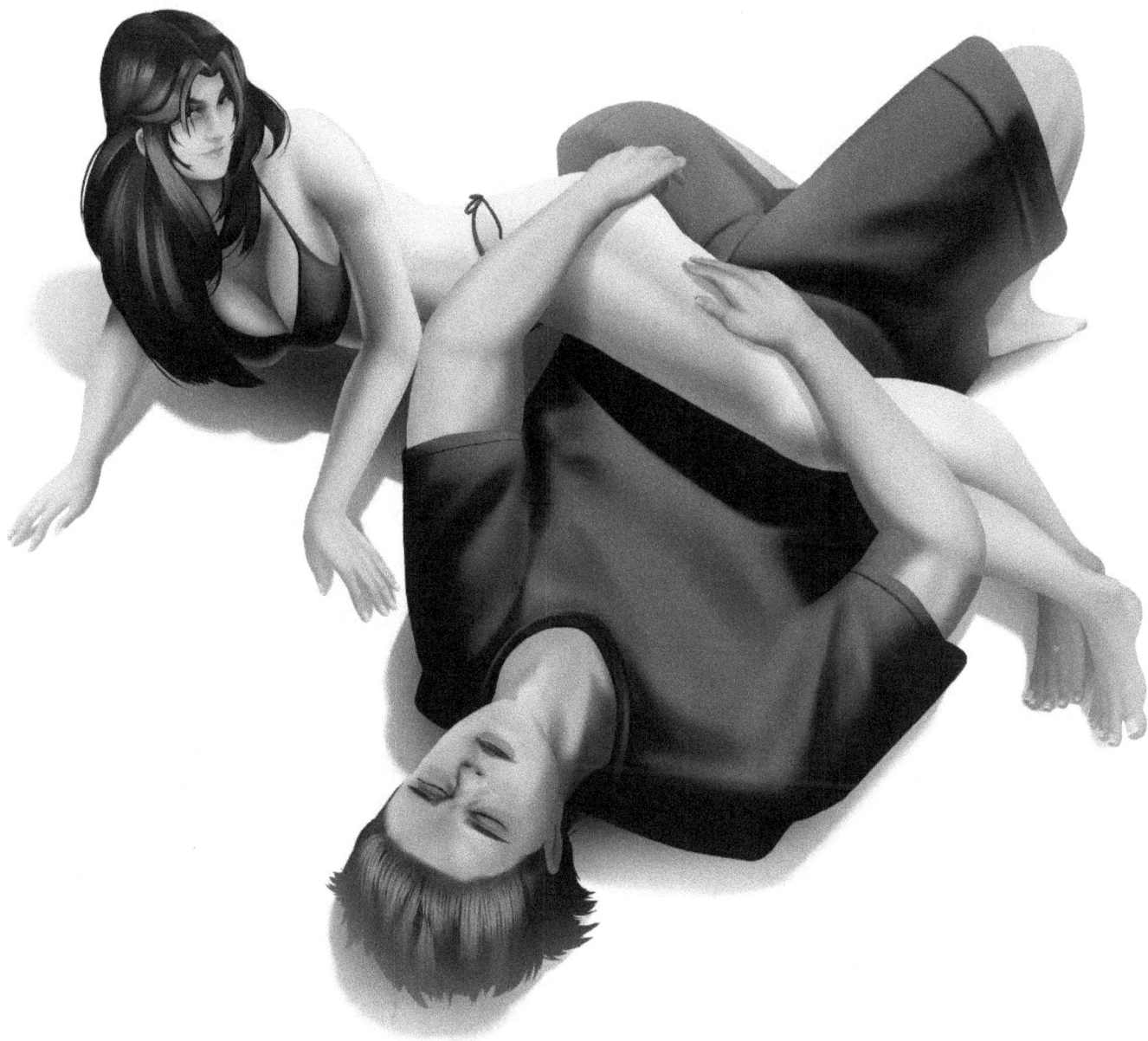

**Reverse Bodyscissors**. In a reverse bodyscissors, the woman faces away from the man or towards his feet and uses her legs to squeeze his torso.

**Spider Scissor.** The spider scissor is a position similar to the figure four. In this position the female crosses her ankles and attempts to pull her feet to her butt with the victim's head between her legs. A key detail here is that the woman lays slightly beneath the man on her back, and his face and vision get smothered by her calf or calves. This can be a more advanced hold to pull off.

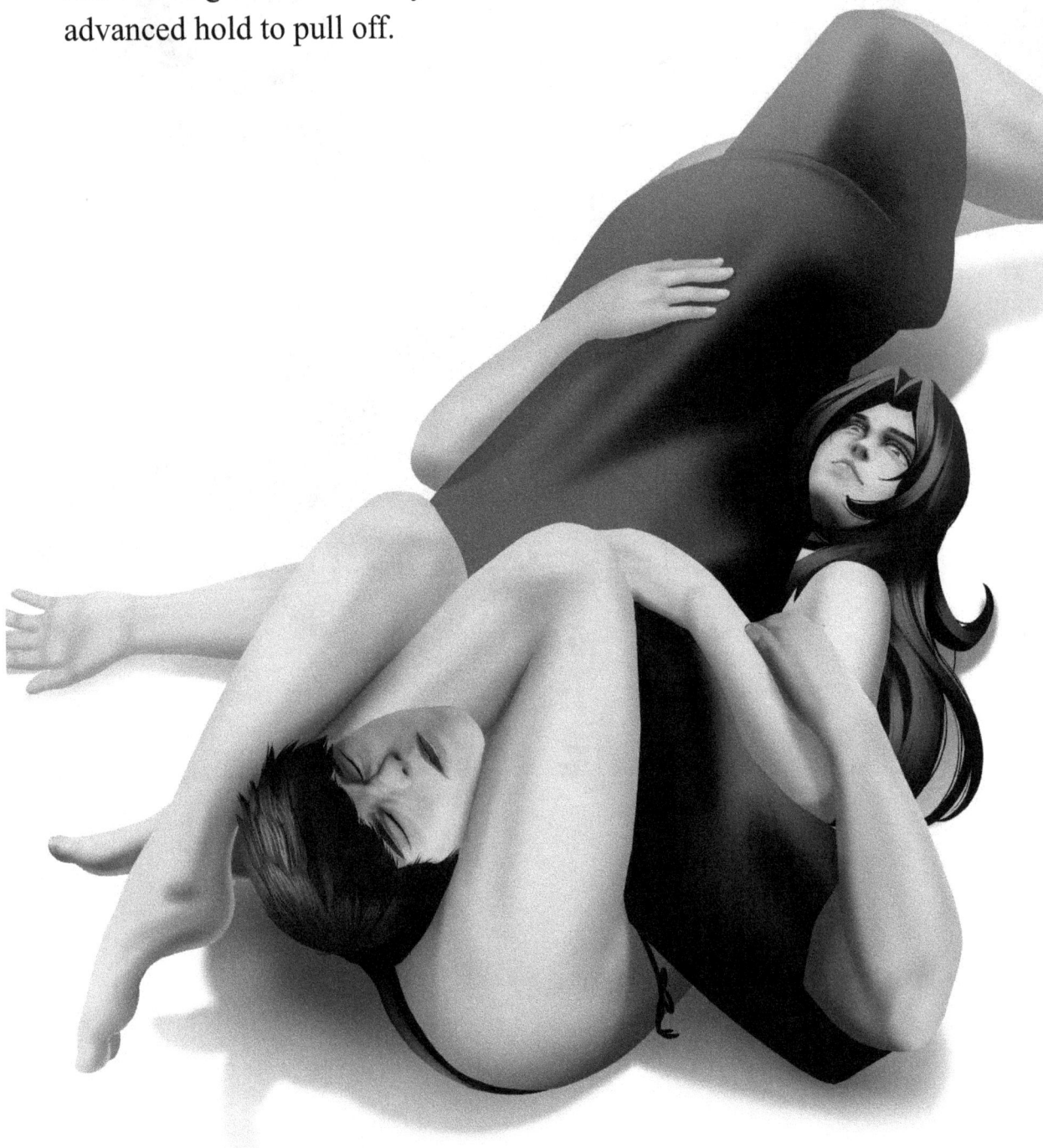

Next up is the **Cradle**. The cradle is a unique hybrid between the infamous side-reverse headscissor and a figure four except the foot isn't pulled all the way back to create the extreme pressure a figure four is known for. It can be considered a variation of either, but the main thing to note is that the legs form a '9' shape.

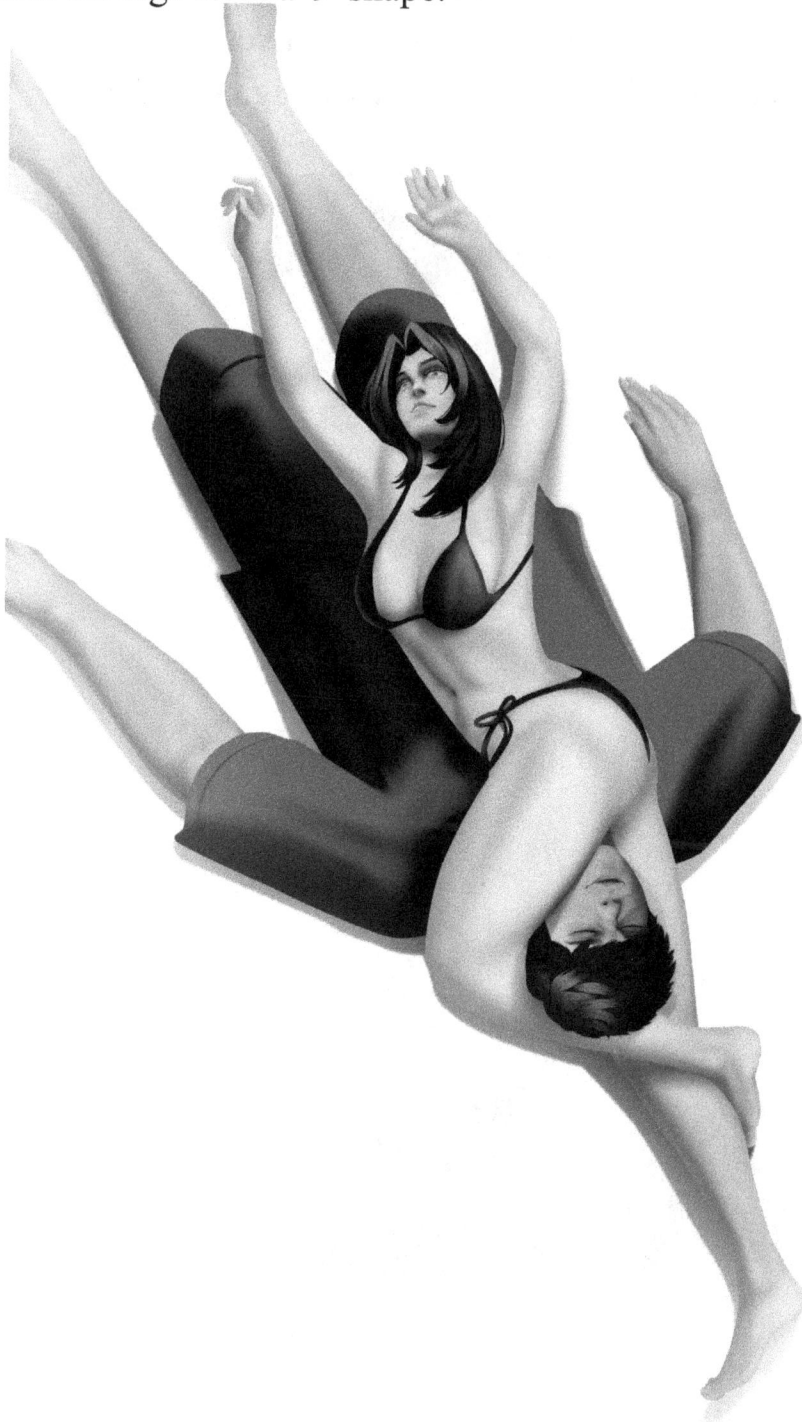

**Foot Scissor.** A broad and wide type of scissor, the foot scissor is simple to think of and easy to apply. It simply is taking both feet and mashing them together at the soles with the victim's head or neck in between. Obviously, this can be done in a plethora of positions that unfortunately won't be defined here.

**Calf Scissor.** It is exactly what you think it is. Once again the almighty, powerful thighs can take a break. A calf scissor is any hold where the neck or head is squeezed solely between two calves. Similar to the foot scissor, but not nearly as inescapable as a thigh based hold.

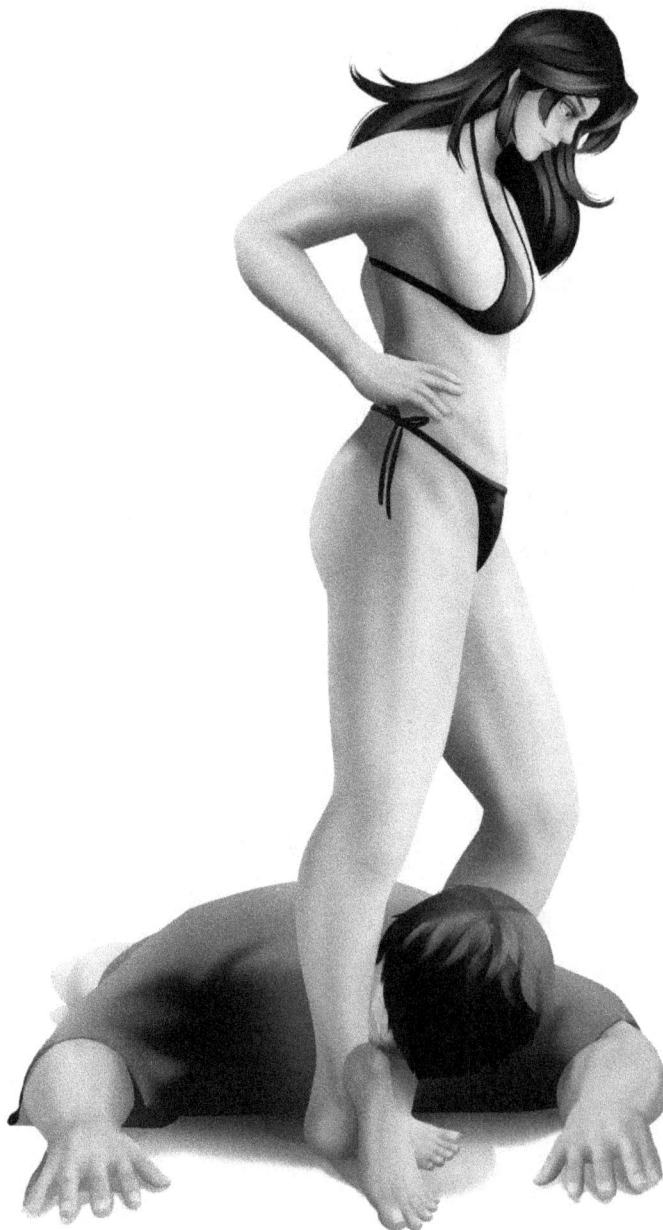

**Thighjob**. Lastly, but definitely not least, is the controversial thighjob or any type of legjob. Some will argue this technically falls under the bodyscissor category while others will argue this is a valid headscissor hold because there is indeed a head trapped. To put it bluntly, a thighjob is where the man's penis is trapped between the thighs of the woman. She squeezes her glutes, grinds strokes, wiggles, and jiggles on the penis until it ultimately submits to the soft and smooth power of her legs. In knowing that it really can be more of a combination of a thigh and ass job due to the extreme power the glutes will have over the experience in certain positions. It is highly advised though, to be much more sensitive and not to squeeze with even a fraction of the total strength during a thighjob since the head is that of a penis not an actual man.

Of course, there always could be some differences in thighjob ease/satisfaction based on compatibility with your partner. For example, if the woman has mega-thighs bigger than a watermelon or if the man has a penis that is too short to make it all the way through her thighs, problems could arise. By no means does that remove your ability to enjoy a thighjob, but the visual aspect of a thighjob where one partner (or both) can view the live results of the woman's hard work won't be something you get to experience. This is mainly because the thighs will completely devour the penis, swallowing it whole and removing it from any view. She can still conquer his penis, but the entirety of the violently resisted and explosive submission will be concealed between her legs.

But don't worry! Some types might or might not work for everyone. There are multiple variations of the thighjob such as the **Reverse Thighjob** where the man watches the woman's glutes squeeze out his essence from just behind her feet, the **Kissing Thighjob** where the woman lays on the man's stomach in a position where they can easily kiss each other, and the **Calf or Footjobs** where her thighs aren't even the main antagonist of the story at all, rather a background character!

Heart-wrenching Reverse Thighjob:

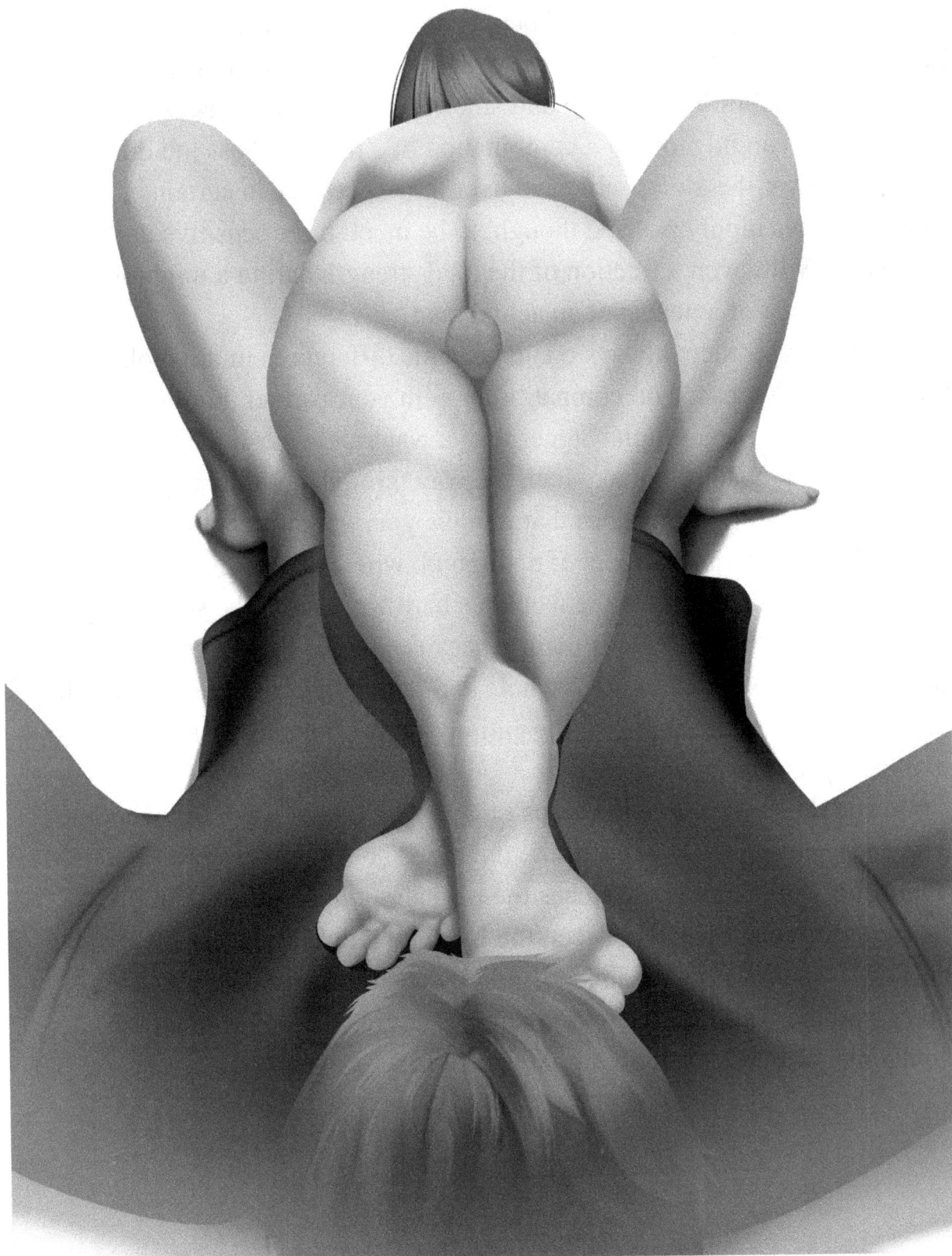

Stimulating Kissing Thighjob:

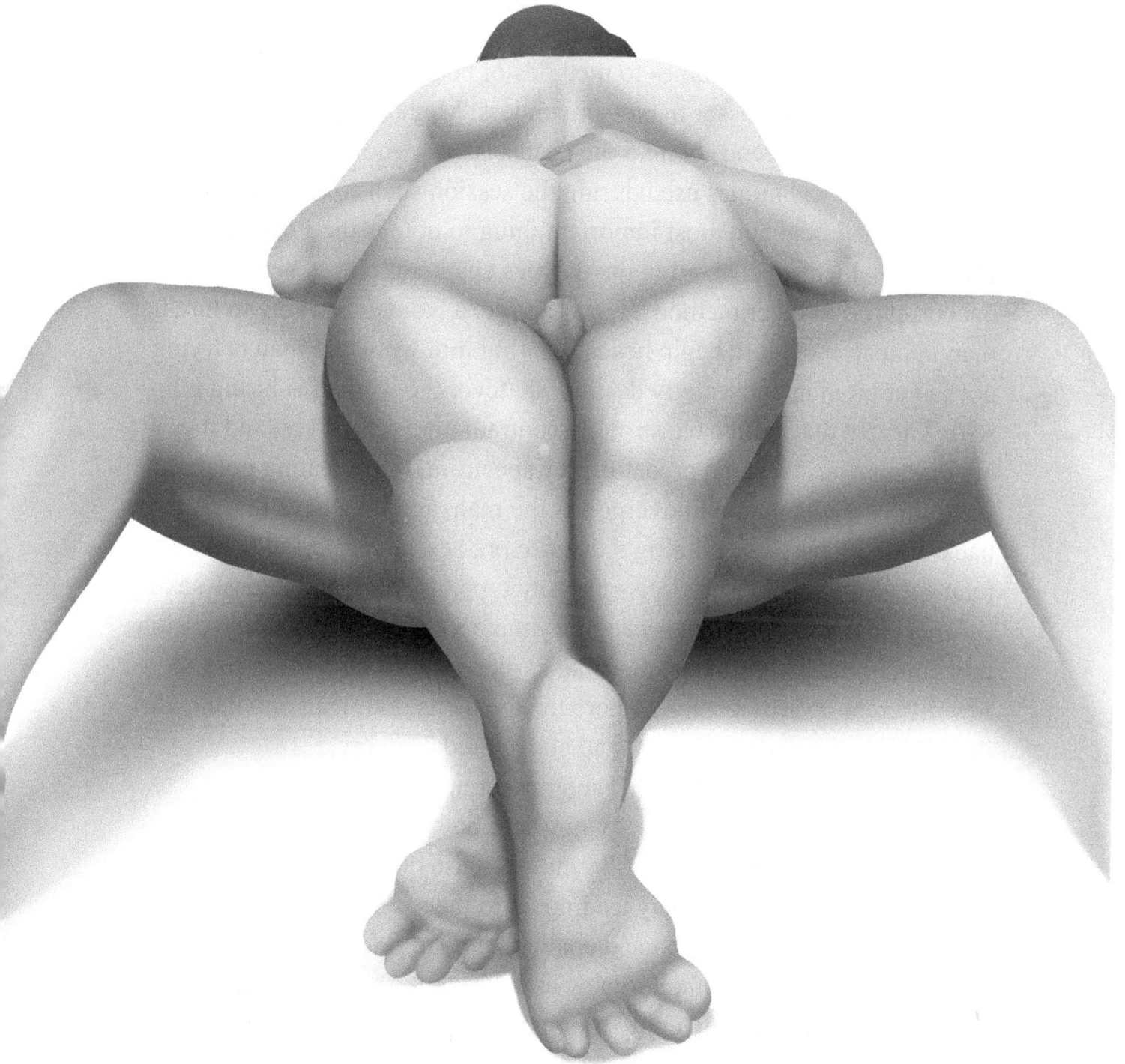

# Chapter 7

## Methods of Headscissoring

While the types were plentiful and varied, different methods or 'games' and techniques involving headscissors can be equally mind-blowing. When it comes to methods of headscissoring, the type or position of the headscissor matters much less. Methods typically focus more on a hidden agenda behind the headscissor session itself. They also can be special techniques used during the session such as the guillotine method. The initial and most important thing to note is the **Polarity Dynamic** which we covered in the degrees chapter. Polarity sets the backdrop for all other methods. For example, a woman is trying to lure her man in close enough to begin headscissoring him while the man is trying not to get lured in but secretly desires whatever the woman is luring him with. Clearly they both have strongly contradicting objectives, and they are on opposite sides of a predator/prey spectrum, thus creating polarity. Eventually the woman will overpower the man, and they have this on the back of their conscience during the entire pre-session or period before the man gets caught in her headscissors. Any type of strong and intense sexual polarity falls into this category and can make a simple headscissor session much more intense without squeezing harder at all or increasing risk. A few different polarity combos where the female is dominant and the male is submissive include: as mentioned above predator/prey, champion/challenger, queen/serf, and master/apprentice or slave.

Not only does a clear role-play where both parties select a submissive or dominant role to slip into increase polarity for the whole session, dirty talk and foreplay leading up to the session are now easier to complete. Take the champion and challenger combo for example. Previously, the extent of the foreplay and dirty talk/sexting before the session was, "I'm going to enjoy trapping you between my thighs tomorrow night." Now with utilizing a polarity dynamic (challenger/champion), it can be more like, "Tomorrow night I am going to finally defeat you and crown myself the champion." Followed by, "Do you really think you have what it takes to defeat me? Every single challenger has begged for mercy while squirming between my thighs…you will be no different." and so forth. Polarity is incredibly important in the bedroom outside of headscissoring, and when brought into headscissoring the sessions do get more complicated. It should be brought in regardless of how strange it is at first because in the long run the experiences will also get more rewarding.

The first actual method to spice up a headscissor session involves breath play, like most headscissors. It has been referred to as the horrific *Anaconda Method*. Simple in theory to pull off and following the polarity rule, it starts with a woman wanting to put the man in her headscissor. His goal, however, is to escape or prevent being caught in her headscissors. Similar to a predator/prey dynamic. Her thighs are to be inescapable yet hypnotizingly desirable. The act of luring in the male despite her dangerous and predatory legs can up the stimulation for both parties and even become a game in and of itself due to its intense sexual polarity. If luring in her prey fails, the woman can simply take a more aggressive predator playstyle, catching her man and forcing him in between her legs against his will (consensual nonconsent). Once caught by either method, there sometimes may be lots of fighting to keep him subdued and in the hold. Perhaps he will enjoy the bliss of her beauty and not attempt to escape. It all depends on the dynamic the couple has or wants. However, once he gets caught the woman starts to play the real game with her prey.

With every breath the male exhales, ever so slightly she constricts her thighs around his throat like a massive anaconda. It should be such a miniscule change that the victim fails to even recognize what is happening for several breaths. This can be very difficult to pull off if she isn't paying careful attention to his inhales and exhales. Of course, practice can make her better at detecting his breath over time. Eventually, the male will realize that every time he exhales more pressure is applied. This is when the real struggle begins, and sensations and emotions drastically increase.

The panic and sexualized fear that sets in can be euphoric whether you are experiencing it or forcing it upon your partner. Escape isn't an option because chances are he has desperately tried that already. Begging isn't an option, the woman has him exactly where she wants him and maybe even where he belongs. Air quickly becomes a scarce resource because her soft thighs slowly clench down on him with each breath. The only outcome for the man is defeat. The fear of whatever that means for the individual session will make his heart skip as he looks his loving partner in the eyes (if the position permits). The woman of course gets to watch him panic with each breath he takes knowing sooner than later he will be hers.

Depending on how thirsty her prey is for air and how much pressure she adds with each breath, this method can take minutes up to half an hour to complete, but the outcome is always the same. Here the scissor can be taken to the fifth or sixth degree, ending in a tap out submission or a full blown knock out. Either way the inevitable is a slow and drawn out experience that builds insane amounts of anticipation, fear, and pleasure. The prolonged submission gives both parties plenty of time to dirty talk and tease. This can be an amazing foreplay before other types of sex for obvious, heart-throbbing reasons.

Very similar to the anaconda method, the *Python Method* is equally heart wrenching. All of the rules are the exact same as the anaconda method, but instead of squeezing only when the man exhales, the woman must ever so slightly tighten the grip her legs have on the man's neck, indefinitely. It doesn't matter if he is breathing or holding his breath, once she catches him with her legs she will constrict them tighter around him as slowly as she possibly can until his demise is upon him.

Mentioned beforehand in Chapter 5, the *Squeeze for Slurp Method* is a great low-risk game to play. It can be started by thigh worship or straight up going down on the woman. The rules are even easier than the previous method's rules, for roughly every second the male is squeezed in a headscissor one lick or kiss must be given to the woman's lips of life. These kisses aren't pecks either. They should be long and drawn out. This can be used as a type of foreplay until the real oral sex starts, cunnilingus without worrying about any distracting headscissoring, or it can be the main course as well.

Speaking of cunnilingus, the ***Cunnilingus Method*** is unsurprisingly similar. The male, goes down on the female until she is sufficiently satisfied. When she is satisfied with his tongue work, she makes it clear by putting him in a headscissor. This can take five minutes, or this can take over an hour. As the man, your focus is her pleasure. Do your homework, and learn how to go down on her. As the woman, your focus is… your pleasure…until your pleasure has been satiated. After she is satisfied enough to focus on the man's pleasure, those beautiful thighs will slowly yet methodically or abruptly and violently clamp down on his neck starting the headscissor session, focusing on his pleasure, and ending the cunnilingus.

One variation is the ***Squirt for Squeeze Method***. Here, the rules are nice and easy. If the female squirts, she headscissors the male. How long? Up to you.

The fabled ***Facesit Worship*** is a fantastic combo between the reverse headscissor and the reverse facesit. Tie in some body worship and the combo becomes a finishing method. It can start either in a reverse headscissor or the reverse facesit, but the male, if not being smothered or squeezed out, is required to kiss and lick the ass, thighs, or pussy that his mouth can reach, indefinitely. If the squeeze pressure or ass smothering is too much for him he can tap, and the woman gives him a bit of mercy in the form of immediate time to gasp for air and worship her with his kisses. If he taps three times, the woman swaps positions. For example, if she was reverse facesitting him when he tapped a third time…boom! A swift scoop between the thighs and now it's a reverse headscissor. He is still required to kiss away if she isn't squeezing!

Lastly, I wanted to provide some advice for reverse facesitting that can be applied anytime outside of this method. While this tiny, little nugget of information may not help too much, it is interesting enough for me to include. When in a reverse facesitting position with the female's thighs acting as earmuffs for her victim, she can increase pleasure for both parties. If she is flexible enough, she can slip her feet under the back of the male's head to provide an even higher level of closeness for him as well as more control over him. With the toes of her opposite feet barely touching each other, she can use her feet that are cusping the back of the man's head to lift him up further into her butt at will. For him it will be the final straw. *"She had me where I thought she wanted me…then she scooped me up with her feet and shoved me further in without even using her hands. I'm in love. I can't escape."*

(Please note, this quote is predicted and not guaranteed to happen in real life if this technique is used.)

Now, it is necessary to please the female partner, but if they want to make a headscissor session even better for the male's stimulation there are a few oral options to up the ante. The best position for oral sex which focuses on the man would have to be the reverse headscissor, just another reason it is a top tier if not the best hold. Thus, the ***Reverse Headscissor Blow Job*** and its following variations are heart throbbing methods. The reverse headscissor blow job is exactly what it sounds like: a blow job, while the man is in a reverse headscissor. That alone can be experimented with the different degrees and such. With it being a simple concept, let's skip over it and get straight into a couple of the variations.

The suspense building ***Ejaculation = KO Method*** will get the blood flowing through every man. Butterflies will flutter in any man's stomach once he realizes the rules. Trapped in a third degree headscissor, he gets to view the ass of his partner and enjoy the oral sex she provides at the same time! Being unable to escape the hold, it becomes a battle of attrition. If---when he ejaculates, those lovely, lady legs he so daringly loves slowly get to work and put him to sleep, instantly turning it into a sixth degree headscissor.

A less frightening and suspenseful variation is the ***Tap Out to Max Out Method***. While going down on the man trapped in her reverse headscissor, the woman is always doing one of two things: squeezing his head/neck or sucking his penis. If he taps while she is sucking him, in an attempt to hold on to his load a little bit longer, she obliges and shows his penis mercy. The tradeoff? She begins applying pressure to his head instead. Then when in preference to getting knocked out, he taps again, she obliges and shows his head mercy. However, now she gets back to applying the pressure to his tiny head. In the end his demise is inevitable. She will always conquer him either by knocking him out with her man mashing thighs or by draining him of his life essence with her soft, wet lips.

There is always inherent danger during a blow job. That danger is ejaculation, which can be viewed as the ultimate form of submission to a woman. With the **Last Stand Method** the majority of pressure is saved for the end to ensure this danger comes to bursting fruition. The third degree headscissor seems safe, but whenever the male feels as though his penis is nearing the end of its life (ejaculation is approaching if not imminent) he taps. This communicates to his woman he is about to finish. In response she immediately squeezes the scissor tightly and begins whatever 'finishing' oral method she likes to use the most. She doesn't let go of the squeeze until he ejaculates (or passes out), and after he is drained she is free to headscissor him all she wants, if she wants.

Next up there is something I like to call **Contract and Jac**. Like the previous few this is best done in a reverse headscissor with oral, but oral nor the reverse position are required. The woman brings the man to orgasm, and immediately changes her rhythmic motions to match the contractions of his orgasm…specifically her legs. At his first explosive release she stops squeezing her legs together completely, and then between the pulses she squeezes him firmly with her thighs. This will start off with intensity due to the quick stop and start squeezing, but as the man's ejaculation slowly subsides the length of each squeeze increases. Basically, if the woman sees sperm coming out of his penis she won't grip him with her legs. This can be taken to a knock out or a tap out.

84

In addition to all of the oral methods, most of which are mostly only possible in the reverse headscissor hold, there also is the ***Hand Job Method***. As simple as it sounds, the man is in a headscissor while receiving a hand job. This method can happen in more types/holds than a blow job method could, especially if the female is flexible or has long arms and legs. One of the best positions to try this in is the front headscissor where the woman can watch the man's face. This will increase the intensity of the act due to intimate eye contact.

The ***Lotion Method*** is a soft and playful experience. It is very simple to understand and execute, although it may take some practice for the woman to get really good at it. Firstly, the man lathers lotion all over the woman's legs, mainly on her inner thighs and inner calves. He makes sure to use excess lotion, and then he does it a second time. Once the woman's legs are overly lotioned by quite a bit, she applies the lotion to the man's head. She can only use her legs, which have plenty of lubricant to spare, in her efforts to lube up her man. This is why he made sure to apply extra lotion to her inner thighs. Her inner thighs will smother him for as long as it takes to dry up the lotion, and they are typically what will be able to do most of the work most easily. For added polarity, the man can try to escape or resist her attempts at applying the lotion, and if extra intensity is desired some bondage or handcuffs for him after he has applied lotion to her legs will make the struggle even more heart throbbing.

Then we have the ***Guillotine Method.*** As the name suggests it does involve a fair bit of pain. However, this acts better as a technique than a method. The woman scoops up her man in a front facing side headscissor, reverse side headscissor, or side headscissor (hopefully not the latter). She then chops away at his neck or head by lifting the top leg straight up into the sky as far as it can go and forcing it back into the locked position as quickly as possible. If the pain a falling leg causes for the neck isn't enough, she can lock the position and immediately squeeze for extra damage.

Taking a break from the pain again, **Cuddle Headscissors** are a much softer method to apply. Mentioned multiple times before, this is simply when two partners cuddle in a headscissor. The degree can vary slightly, but squeezy truly is not the main focus of this method. The importance of this method is simply to feel close to one another in a headscissor. Obviously, the male is going to experience the headscissor much differently, but if KO's or tap outs become the main focus instead of bonding time together it is no longer just cuddling and is now a full blown headscissor session. Nothing is wrong with this change, but it must be noted. In addition, try not to fall asleep while cuddling in a headscissor, male or female. This can be a safety risk.

**Killer Cuddles** are a variant of normal cuddle headscissors. The method starts in a normal cuddle position absent of any headscissoring (unless bodyscissoring in the form of her legs around his waist). The head is free, and the partners may kiss or move relatively freely. The spicy part is…the male isn't allowed to leave the cuddle, and whenever the female wants she can aggressively surprise attack her man and scoop him up in a headscissor to start a headscissor session. It is called killer cuddles because that outcome is GUARANTEED. It isn't a matter of if, rather when. She can use her lips, hands, or even her legs to build suspense. The man is not allowed to leave the bed even if she does. He can resist her attempts at putting him in a headscissor if he chooses, but since he is not allowed to leave the bed she eventually will capture him and wreak havoc.

Don't get too excited to cuddle because with the **Challenge Reverse BJ** method the killer cuddles method becomes an intense game for survival. With all of the understood rules of the killer cuddle some added zest is provided. When the female is ready to start the headscissor session, she starts a stopwatch on her phone. Immediately afterwards she has two extremely time sensitive goals. First, catch the man in a reverse headscissor despite any resistance he may fight back with. Second, give him a blowjob where he finishes as fast as possible. The stopwatch is set to see how quickly she can conquer the male, from the first attempt of catching him between her thighs up until the first throbbing pulse of submission fluttering between her lips, time is ticking. Can she get a new record? Can he set a new record for survival time? How long do you think you would last?

Next we have good ole' **Body Worship**. Yep, that's it. The male kisses and licks the thighs, legs, ass, and groin to the woman's content. She can point at a part of her body, and his lips must land there as quickly as possible until she points again. She can squeeze his head between her legs, but the worship must resume feverishly if and when she releases him from her vice grip.

**Silent Scissors.** Silent scissors is a method that could increase pleasure for just about every dynamic. The concept of this method is that the man is not allowed to speak to the woman with the obvious exception of the safe word. The extent of what he isn't allowed to say can vary. For example in a sadistic type of session, if he mutters a single word he could risk immediate punishment. Whereas in a playful session the woman may allow him to beg her: mercy, please, babe, etc. She can even let him speak a full sentence before squeezing him silent once more. The amount he can get away with is up to the woman, and how much she lets him get away with combined with how she punishes him and taunts him for speaking can change the dynamic greatly.

A classic: **Mixed Wrestling**. Nervous? I would be. Both partners wrestle each other, either nude, clothed, or even oiled. If the female wins or even manages to pin her partner one time, what once was a wrestling session now is a headscissor session. Good luck coming out on top of that one! If the female loses…well maybe the male wants to dominate that night. It could go either way, but if one partner is way stronger or knows martial arts or wrestling of any form to a considerable level…they both know how it's going to end. Also, it isn't wrong if the parties agree who is going to win beforehand. For example, if the male and the female both want a headscissor outcome, but the male is a black belt in Jiu Jitsu they can agree to let the female win. There is nothing wrong with fake wrestling in the intimacy of your relationship.

A variant of mixed wrestling, rather the more intense sequel: **Bondage Wrestling**. Even more heart fluttering, I would be more than nervous as well. It's okay! Here the goal isn't simply to subdue and procure a tap or knockout from the opponent. Your goal is to tie them up to the point they can't untie themself. At that point, as agreed upon prior to starting a bondage wrestling session, you can have your way with them. A good way to play this out is to have about three or four extra bondage ropes to use on the ground around you and your partner. In addition to that, use another rope to tie around each of your wrists. This way at any point a dangling rope is hanging from both you and your partner's wrists. This rope can be used against the person it dangles from. Of course, once the female wraps up the male she can have a headscissor session with him, but be advised in any position where the male is unable to tap she should pay extra attention to his state of consciousness at all times. Regardless, the male doesn't even need to be tied up to be eligible for her headscissors. The woman can headscissor him to make tying her victim up easier. Personally, I wouldn't be too focused on what my arm is being tied to if I can't breathe between a pair of thighs. Also, the headscissor may physically make it impossible for the male to prevent the female's actions, by restraint alone! Everything is all up to the parties at play, and the fear of losing has warranted risk behind it!

Now let's take some time to talk about an interesting game-like method, **Fold or Five**. This method is heavy in polarity dynamics which put the woman in the dominant position...outside of the bedroom. Let's look at a couple who are playing this game. The couple knows they are going to have sex later in the night, specifically a headscissor session, but they are going out on a date first. If playing fold or five, the woman gets twelve demands that she can force on her man throughout the date night. The man gets only two options for each of her demands: fold or five. Those are the only two outcomes.

For example, the couple go hiking down a trail before dinner. After some time they are completely alone. The woman says, "Fold or five. Get down on your knees and start kissing my ass passionately until I tell you to stop." The woman is demanding something from her partner. The man can either fold and obey her, risking getting caught in public kissing her butt, or the man can disobey her and take five. Five being five full minutes of unknown degree headscissoring after the date night. As discussed in Chapter 3, the unknown degree is when the man has no clue how intense the headscissor session will be. The woman has full control over whether or not he will be knocked out, forced to tap out, or even squeezed at all.

The fact that the woman gets twelve different demands means that if the man refuses to do what she asks all twelve times, he is subject to a full **hour** of headscissoring at her mercy later that night as punishment for disobeying her. This dynamic can be experimented with every single date night, and due to its unpredictability not one game of fold or five will ever be the exact same as another...nor will the punishment headscissors.

The last of our inconclusive list is ***Public Headscissoring***. This method plays a bit on the humiliation aspect of headscissoring as well as any exhibitionism desires either party may have. All that one must do is be outside when the headscissor session occurs. Obviously, wearing clothes is a great idea if you choose to do this. Sometimes, if someone sees a man getting squeezed out between a woman's thighs they will ignore it completely or ask if the woman is okay. When they notice that she is fine and in complete control they may even congratulate her or praise her for her independence and dominance. If the humiliation aspect is absent in either party, this is just funny because chances are the male asked for it. That however, does not mean all encounters will be like that.

Avoid places where people may be. Safety is not guaranteed outside, and law enforcement might get involved, especially if it is intense headscissoring or perceived as sexual in any way. Also, think about the kids! Do you want them to see it? If not, and hopefully not, be more discreet indoors or find a more secluded spot outside. However, I understand that nature and headscissors are a beautiful combination! I completely agree with the multiple desires to have a session outside. So here are some thought provoking locations to headscissor in the insafety of the outdoors: A beach, in the forest, on a mountain, in a field, under a bridge, in your backyard, in your fenced in backyard, in your fenced in backyard at night where nobody can see you, by the lake, under the moon (again all of these ideally at night), camping near the Grand Canyon, in the desert, on a rarely used hiking trail, or even on a trampoline.

The list goes on and on, but my biggest two concerns for anyone trying outside headscissoring is the chance of being caught by other humans followed by the chance a natural predator decides to investigate, examples include a bear or mountain lion. For the former, in most cases, any humans concerned about your situation typically can be dismissed by the woman if she says, "Oh sorry! Yes, I'm fine. I was just reminding my boyfriend why I'm always right." This or some other variant that makes the male look like he deserves the headscissoring but not handcuffs should remove any and all concerns for most investigative pedestrians if the headscissors themselves aren't too intense. *Most.* As for the animals, anything that would protect you from them if encountered in the wild would be recommended to have. It doesn't help that one of the woman's strongest allies could be resting unconscious between her inescapable legs if an animal did decide to attack. Stay safe out there and enjoy the scenery.

That is the full list of methods I have compiled, and there are many more to discover and create. The movement and placement of body parts with a good sexual power dynamic working behind the scenes makes for great methods. There is still one thing lacking. Teasing. The first fraction of teasing that I will talk about is unpredictability. When a man is being headscissored without knowing what will happen next the anxiety and anticipation can add to the excitement and enjoyment for everyone involved. In addition to that, it also removes a sense of control from him and gives it to the woman. He has no clue what she is about to do. A good example of this can be _setting and breaking the pattern_. This is where the woman creates a cycle of rhythmic movements that the man learns and expects before completely breaking the pattern with something unpredictable. For example:

- In a standing reverse headscissor, the woman holds the man close without squeezing and sways her hips from the left to the right, pulling the man's head back and forth gently.
- After several seconds she stops swaying and begins contracting her glute and thigh muscles rapidly to create soft, pulsing squeezes on him.
- After several more seconds she abruptly squeezes tight and hard for another seven seconds.
- Then she returns to the swaying and repeats the pattern multiple times.
- Eventually, she breaks the pattern by abruptly squeezing tighter and tighter during the middle of the swaying. This will catch the man off guard as he thought he was safe until after the pulses. From here she can create a new pattern for him to learn, or even return to the previous pattern. Either way he will still feel much less in control since the pattern he learned to expect has already been broken once. This can be very fun for everyone involved.

Sexual teasing in the form of unpredictability isn't exclusive to headscissoring either. It can be done in any sexual situation, and is extremely easy to do. Setting and breaking a pattern isn't necessary either; that is just a good way to practice being unpredictable. As long as the partner who is not in control has no clue what is going to happen next (ex: sway to the right, stroke deep, fast, slow, grip tight, kiss, etc.) the dominant is creating a beautifully unpredictable environment for their submissive.

Now, we get to another section of teasing. In an attempt to guide you in uplifting the experience, I will provide a list of things that could be said before, during, or after a headscissor session to increase pleasure. These starter phrases aren't in chronological order. Some of them can be used together, and some of them work better for different types of power dynamics and desires. Obviously, you can edit anything to better suit your needs. First up we have some things that could be said before the session:

Male, "Your legs look so soft."

Male, "Do you really think your legs could catch me?"

Female, "My thighs are so lonely…they miss your warmth."

Male, "I'd escape with no problem."

Female, "I think my legs need some attention…"

Female, "My thighs are getting a little hungry for you…"

Male. "I owe you a couple leg kisses…"

Male, "I'd like to see you try to put me in my place."

Female, "Your place is trapped between my legs. I can put you there with ease."

Female, "I love you."

Female, "You're packing to stay the night right? Because once my legs catch you…you won't be going anywhere…"

Male, "Do you think I could escape your thighs?"

Female, "I can't wait for you to get here. They are shaved, silky smooth, warm, soft, and patiently waiting for their prey…"

Male, "What will happen when I get there?"

Male, "The battle will be incredible."

Male, "When was the last time we had a duel again? And remember who won?"

Female, "When you get here my legs will…well let's just say they are very excited to play with you…"

Female, "You would be the only one to defeat me…my thighs have slain dozens before you."

Male, "You call your legs man-mashers? Is that a joke?"

Female, "You're going to learn why my thighs are called man-mashers."

Female, "Once caught by my thighs…I will make you beg."

Male, "I have a bottle of lotion for you…"

Female, "Ooh…should I let you lather me with it before or after I conquer you?"

Male, "I love you."

Male, "Your legs are hypnotizing me."

Male, "What are you going to do to me with them?"

Female, "My legs are very alluring are they not? You should come a little closer to them."

Female, "How long do you think you're going to last once I catch you?"

Male, "I am willing to sacrifice myself for the greater good!"

Female, "You're freezing! Let me warm you up…my thighs can melt away your stress!"

Female, "Just let them catch you…I'll let you squeeze my butt like a stress ball if you want."

Female, Unsolicited sext of legs in leggings hours before meeting up. "They miss you…"

During the session the female will do most of the talking since the male might be too out of breath to tease verbally. Here is the list of some starter phrases to use during the headscissor session:

Female, "Finally! I didn't think it would take this long to catch you."

Female, "Stop fighting! It's over, baby. They've caught you."

Male, "Uh oh! Oh no! Shit!"

Female, "And just like that…how do they feel around your neck? Sooooo snug…"

Female, "Now that I've caught you, let's have some fun shall we?"

Male, "I can still escape!"

Male, "How did you do that?! You just scooped me up and caught me so easily!"

Female, "I love you."

Female, "My legs look so much better with you trapped between them. Can I take a photo…or five?"

Female, "You're not in control anymore, so you're going to do as I say. Understand?"

Male, "Baby please!"

Male, "Have mercy!"

Female, "Enjoying the view?"

Female, "Start kissing or I start squeezing."

Female, "Go ahead and prove to me how beautiful I am. Show me you love me."

Male, "I LOVE you."

Male, "They are so soft...so so tight...inescapable."

Male, "I'll never surrender!"

Male, "Baby you win you win! You own me!"

Female, "Aww, I think I'm going to start squeezing."

Female, "My thighs feel so warm and comforting...don't they?"

Female, "I told you that I'd win. My legs already caught you. You didn't stand a chance."

Female, "Any final words before I finish you?"

Female, "Nice and tight..."

Female, "You are so cute when you squirm..."

Female, "This is where you'll be all night."

Female, "How many squeezes do you think I can do in a minute?"

Female, "Try to escape. Go ahead...try."

Female, "It's just you and my legs...let their warmth melt away all...your...worries."

Female, "Breathe for me. Aw you can't?"

Male, "I don't think I'm gonna escape."

Female, "You're not going to escape. My legs always finish my prey..."

Female, "I want to practice some combos. Tell me which one leaves you the weakest."

Female, "Shhhh...I know baby...it's nice and tight..."

Female, "Give in to my grip..."

Female, "Can I keep you here forever?"

Male, "Can I stay here forever?"

Female, "Time for my finishing move."

Female, "You just couldn't resist my legs could you? I don't blame you...they always get me what I want..."

Female, "Wake up. You just got mashed by my man mashers...do you still think it's funny to call them that?"

Lastly we have some phrases to use after the session. Like all of the phrases, they don't necessarily connect with any other phrases, can be edited to suit your needs, and are starter phrases to help you begin or practice a teasing arc or dialogue. Get creative and think of your own teases that you would like to use or hear during a session. Here is my post-session starter phrase list:

Female, "That made me feel so powerful, I didn't go too hard on you did I?"
Male, "When you did X I genuinely thought you were going to finish me."
Male, "I love you."
Female, "You liked my unpredictability didn't you?"
Male, "Holy shit…I was at your mercy!"
Male, "I didn't escape…"
Female, "Better luck next time baby."
Female, "You put up a good fight."
Female, "I really liked it when you X"
Male, "Oh my! Stop moving and stroking them like they are innocent!"
Male, "Does this mean I lost?"
Female, "Next time I'm not letting you go."
Female, "Come here!" Open armed, open legged, kissy face inviting male to get caught in her embrace where she will wrap all her limbs around him before kissing on him and cuddling him indefinitely (a form of aftercare).
Female, "You said you were going to defeat me?"
Female, "What did you think of my finisher?"
Male, "That combo literally left me weak."
Female, "Now that I've conquered you with my legs…it's time I conquer you…with 'her' (referring to her vagina)."
Female, "My legs got to feast on you…but that isn't the only thing that needs fed."
Female, "I love you."
Male, "I loved how you maintained eye contact as you slowly put me to sleep."

Male, "I think your panties might be in the way for what happens next..."

Female, "If you try X again, I will put my panties in your mouth next time."

Female, "My thighs already miss you..."

Male, "That was literally heaven."

Female, "You belong between my legs baby...it feels weird not having you there."

Female, "Just because I let you go doesn't mean we are done in the bedroom..."

Male, "You won...you won baby...you won."

Male, "How can your legs be so soft and tender yet so tight and merciless?"

The post-session phrases are equally about communication as they are teasing. In some cases the session itself is the entire sexual act whereas in other cases the session is the foreplay to something else. In the former, teasing verbally typically doesn't last too long afterwards, but that certainly doesn't mean it can't. In the latter, since this is a transition between acts of sex, teasing verbally is a great idea to help two partners slip into their next act of intimacy while keeping things hot.

# Chapter 8

## Rewards and Risks

There are quite a few rewards and risks to headscissoring that one must weigh before becoming a part of the community. Obviously, the higher degree headscissors will become more and more risky with heavily diminishing returns. For example, a ninth degree headscissor risks jail time, mental trauma, the loss of a partner, and guilt for the female. It nullifies all risks for the male since he got thighed down to death in a Motel 6 bedroom. The rewards? For the female bragging rights that she killed a man with her legs, but that is arbitrary because most people are capable of killing with their legs. For the male? Well, he's dead, it doesn't matter. 0/10 not worth it in the slightest for either party. With that in mind I will continue to list and explain all of the rewards and risks up to an eighth degree headscissor.

## Rewards:

The most obvious reward, sexual satisfaction and arousal. This can be limited to one party but many times both can experience it. The fulfillment of your desire or need is a reward in and of itself.

Trust building comes to mind next. The fact that a man can trust his woman enough to let her squeeze him to the point he falls unconscious is insane. You typically don't do that with strangers and for good reason. The female also builds trust in her partner at the lower degrees because in a fifth degree headscissor the male taps before falling unconscious. This removes some stress the female might have about knocking her partner out. If you can trust your partner enough to headscissor frequently or intensely, you are setting yourself up to have a stronger relationship.

Another relationship improving reward involves strength. As a man, if you allow your female counterpart to headscissor you up to the eighth degree, she gets to witness her strength first hand in a manner she otherwise wouldn't. This is assuming she doesn't wrestle or take part in any martial arts where she may headscissor someone in a non-sexual way. If she knows her own strength is enough to put any man to sleep, an insurmountable boost to her confidence and self-image will occur. Obviously, this is great for both of you. For the male, he gets to experience her strength first hand. Who doesn't like to see their loved ones be strong? Being happy? Being powerful? Well, he will get to bask in the middle of her glory, boosting his perception of her in a positive manner. Obviously, this will also boost her own perception of herself. Everybody wins.

Changing up the sexual polarity can sometimes keep things fresh in the bedroom. This means that if the male is typically dominant, when the female swaps roles in a non-intrusive and agreed upon manner (for example, headscissoring) the relationship may blossom sexually. This freshness can be heightened by uncertainty. For example, the couple agrees to a fifth degree headscissor session, but they cuddle softly until the woman is ready to start headscissoring without warning. The anticipation will keep him coming back for more. Or, instead of agreeing to headscissor at all, have a sexy wrestling match. You don't know who will win. Headscissoring might not even happen if the male wins. Nobody knows who is dominant until it's too late to change it. This all can help the relationship prosper.

.Closeness is also a major reward of headscissoring. While it can be a highly sexual act, some don't find any sexual arousal from headscissoring alone, and even if you do, that doesn't change the closeness. Headscissoring doesn't necessarily need to happen in the bedroom prior to or after sex. It could be just a different form of cuddling your partner with added restrictions on their chances of escape. On the couch watching a show? Scoop his head up with your legs. The worst that can happen is he tries to escape but fails miserably and realizes being close isn't all that bad. Waking up on a lazy Sunday morning together? Scoop him up and stay in bed with him for an extra thirty minutes. Plus, you won't be able to smell his morning breath if he's between your man mashers. Squeezing isn't even required to make it a headscissor. Both of you are sitting on your phones doing nothing? Scoop him up in an inescapable reverse headscissor while you scroll through Tik Tok. Give him his phone and everybody continues what they were doing but much closer together and with better views. Will this turn him on? It certainly can, but that doesn't mean it has to become sexual. It doesn't mean it can't be sexual either.

New things can help your brain and your relationship grow. If you have never done it before, headscissoring can be considered an art to learn. Over time practicing techniques, methods, positioning, and the whole nine yards will stimulate your mind while also stimulating your relationship by the shared experience with your partner. Look at it as a skill to learn, a skill that the one being headscissored in the relationship wants you to learn! That doesn't mean the victim in this circumstance doesn't have to put in any work either. They need to learn how to be headscissored too, and the only way to do that is communicate with the woman and inquire about what she prefers you do while trapped between her thighs.

Those are all of the perks to headscissoring that I could think of. As with almost everything in this book, the list is inconclusive and more could be added. Notice that nearly all of the benefits improve a relationship more than being benefits for the male alone. Sexual satisfaction is listed first because it easily is the most important benefit for the man, but the rest of these rewards can't be discounted. This is another reason I advocate for headscissoring in a relationship instead of session girls or FWB. While those are perfectly viable options for the empty fulfillment of your sexual desires or needs, you miss out on all of the other benefits by doing so.

## Risks:

Physical risks easily top the list. The first four degrees of headscissor have much fewer physical risks, but higher up that changes. In the fifth degree, soreness and popped blood vessels in the eyes can occur if squeezing intensely where the man refuses to tap or fall unconscious. In addition to that, forcing the victim to tap out one hundred times will easily leave soreness in the neck. At the sixth degree, the risk of death, insanely minor, already exists. While the female stops squeezing immediately after the male is knocked unconscious in the sixth degree, inexperienced females may not know when their partner or victim has passed out. This can lead to death in the very rare and most extreme of cases.

In the seventh degree, things continue to get worse physically as repeated headscissors to the point of knockouts can eventually pop veins in the eyes, force a vomit reflex if there isn't enough grace periods, cause dizziness and lightheadedness, pop a blood vessel, and overall make the male feel as though they are dying. There obviously are lots of ways to remediate this such as not eating much before the session and staying hydrated while not over hydrating, but getting knocked out multiple times insures some physical pain. Most of the more intense side effects are rare and only occur if intense, prolonged squeezing happens. In the eighth degree just about every single physical side effect can occur. That doesn't mean that it will in every case, but the chance is always there and heightened whenever safety is disregarded. Since safety being disregarded is what partially defines the eight degree here is an inconclusive list of things that very likely may happen:

- Dizziness
- Lightheadedness
- Weariness
- Fatigue
- Red or purple face
- Muscle spasming (occurs at and after a knockout)
- Popped eye veins
- Popped other veins
- Nosebleeds (squeezing too strong)
- Drastic changes in blood pressure
- Jaw fractures or jaw related injuries (squeeze placement)

- Neck injuries (squeezing too strong)
- Throat injuries (squeezing too strong)
- Broken Trachea (side headscissor)
- Loss of voice (side headscissor)
- Vomiting (extended squeezing after K.O. or male ate too much prior)
- Blood clots
- Collapsed Artery
- Extended Numbness (days following the session)
- Stroke
- Heart Attack
- Brain damage (lack of oxygen)
- Broken ribs (bodyscissors)

This list already is extremely discouraging, and I am positive that I have missed at least a few other possible risks of headscissoring. Some of these can happen at lower degrees like weariness and dizziness while others typically are a telltale sign that you are in the eighth degree and pushing for the ninth such as nosebleeds, vomiting, or broken bones. Some men may actually want to experience the pain of these side effects, and that is perfectly fine as long as their partner is also consensual about it. Don't let this list discourage you or scare you away from headscissoring because in a third even fourth degree headscissor none of these really happen if you are careful enough. The male might get lightheaded or dizzy in a fourth or fifth degree headscissor, but that is a concrete part of headscissoring, which is inherently risky to begin with. If they want a higher degree, they need to accept that there will be pain, and their partner's need to accept what the potential risks may be before agreeing to provide the pain.

When it comes to the risks versus the rewards it is always up to the individuals at play and whether or not they believe the rewards are worth it. For some, the risks may even be a reward in itself such as the pain that comes with headscissoring. For others, the risks may churn stomachs to even think about experiencing or forcing their beloved partner to experience. Whatever your situation is, take this time to go back to the degrees and dynamics chapter and decide, ideally with your partner: *What is the highest degree I'd like to experience, and what is the degree I want to spend most of my headscissor time in? What dynamic sounds the most comforting to me?* Then your partner gets to ask themselves the same question. The variance between your answers is where you and your partner will have to compromise if possible. The following page can be used to help illustrate your own desires.

Partner wanting to or willing to get headscissored:

Highest degree to try: _____

Favorite dynamic to explore: _____

Degree to spend most time in: _____

Partner wanting to or willing to headscissor:

Highest degree to try: _____

Favorite dynamic to explore: _____

Degree to spend most time in: _____

# Chapter 9

## Headscissoring Safety

If you and your partner have agreed to get into headscissoring, this chapter is a must read, especially if neither or only one of you have experienced or given a headscissor before. At the end of this chapter I will give tips and advice for sessions at different degrees if you wish to skip to that. If not I will start my inconclusive public safety announcement.

First and foremost the utmost important thing to keep in mind whenever headscissoring, or partaking in any sexual act for that matter, is communication. I do not mean getting consent to headscissor or be headscissored, although that is an inherent part of communication and is equally important. My focus is on communication during the session with the understanding that consent has already been acquired by both parties. The male, or victim of the headscissors, should be able to easily communicate discomfort. This most likely will be in the form of a tap out since in some positions the thigh ear-muffs will muffle any sound coming in, and the ass of his woman might muffle any verbal requests he may make. To start, a double tap should equate to the ceasing of any squeezing, smothering, or stretching. This is especially important for newer partners getting into headscissoring.

Obviously, many of you may want to take things further by having ignored taps, knock outs, or prevented taps in the form of bondage or restraints. Perfect! You can certainly do that. The message here isn't to force some rule on you or your experience, but rather encourage you and whoever the headscissoring is happening with to communicate properly. Want to get knocked out senseless? Great, but please communicate that with your partner beforehand and be sure you want that. <u>Be sure both you and your partner are conscious and aware of all the possible risks involved with your desired degree of headscissors</u>. This can be an intense act of sex with lots of different potential risks, so understanding is very necessary. If you and your partner have an equal understanding of what is and isn't allowed during your session as well as what the potential risks for both of you are, then the both of you will feel safer. Even if you want to be put to sleep repeatedly, having a communicated safe word or safe motion will ease the stress on your partner, for they know if you truly can't handle it and are at risk for serious injury you could stop them at any time.

Communication isn't exclusive to tapping out and agreeing on which degree of headscissor. It is the fundamental building block for everything else that makes a headscissor session euphoric, let alone the relationship as a whole. Communicate what you liked, what you disliked, and even inquire about your partner's experience. Frequency, technique, position, method, degree, dynamic, length, teasing, reasons, and so forth can all be shared and analyzed to increase the enjoyment for everyone involved. Understand your partner's sexual desires and why they do or don't like certain sexual aspects of this or any other experience. Even learning can fall under communication. Spend time with each other learning how to have better headscissor sessions by watching occasional headscissors videos. You both could see techniques or things that haven't been listed in this book. What if you wanted to try them? Also, maybe the two of you would benefit from recording one of your sessions and watching it back together, explaining what was going through your mind at various moments or things you wish could've happened that might come to fruition next session.

Lastly, while I know that not everyone will listen to the following, I still will write it as a common sense piece of advice. *Your level of sobriety can and will influence your ability to communicate prior to, during, and after a headscissoring session.* Do with that knowledge as you will but don't come to me if things take a turn for the worse when intoxicated.

Now that the biggest safety concern, communication, has been dealt with we can talk about trust. More so for newer headscissor fans and enjoyers, one can build great trust in their partner by experiencing headscissors. Inadvertently building a stronger relationship whilst simultaneously spicing things up sexually, trust can be amazing. Trust is built in the headscissoring sense, when proper communication is practiced. The woman gains trust that if her man can't handle it he will tap or tell her, and the man gains trust that his woman won't take him further down the rabbit hole than he agreed. These are only two examples, but there are plenty. The safety concern comes in for those who are inexperienced and consequently lack the headscissor trust and wisdom. My advice, while not necessary to follow, is to start in the lower degrees of headscissoring until both partners feel comfortable to take things to the next level. Take your time to learn your own strength, whether that be how strong your thighs are or how resilient your carotid arteries are.

The other aspect to trust that must be stated is more prevalent for non-romantic relationships. If you are wanting to get headscissored by somebody that you don't know in the slightest, that is an obvious cause for concern. Can you do it? Certainly, who am I to tell you not to let your dreams become real life dreams as she puts you to sleep between her legs? That doesn't mean the risk is absent. My simple advice is to get to know the woman who is about to physically (possibly mentally and emotionally) break you with her thighs…before…you know…she absolutely conquers you with her thighs. This refers to everything from women of the night to session girls to your own girlfriend if you have one. It doesn't matter who it is, I advise you not to let them headscissor you if you wouldn't want them in your room when you were asleep. Seems easy enough.

Where to do the headscissoring?! A great question that easily could've been in the first chapter. The answer: anywhere you want! I mentioned public headscissoring as a method in the previous chapter, but there are always risks to location. You could be headscissored on the wobbly kitchen table, have it snap, and break your neck on the way down. Or you could be headscissored outside in your backyard garden from noon to three and not have a single bad thing happen, other than the end of the session of course. The point is that headscissoring is inherently dangerous, and the location doesn't change that too much.

If outdoors: avoid highly populated areas, bring some form of self-defense to ward off any curious animals, have a quick excuse in case anybody wonders what you're doing, and most importantly find a place where you feel comfortable and where you feel safe. If indoors: avoid unsturdy objects (no brainer), post up in an open area for the possible flailing, make sure you and your partner are comfortable, and enjoy the privacy of the indoors. The bed or the bedroom floor is always a great starting spot if you don't know where to begin. Whether indoors or outdoors, headscissors can be done almost anywhere, so enjoy the experience wherever you want. Just be conscientious of the safety of your surroundings, the possibility of onlookers, and the stability of your surroundings.

There are a few quick tips I want to smack you with about placement. Headscissoring can hurt. A lot. Improper placement does, not saying it will, have the possibility of causing serious harm if coupled with extreme and extended pressure. To make this quick, the legs can be placed in about three different spots on the victim (excluding bodyscissors). First, tightly around the throat. Second, around the lower half of the head, mainly the jaw. Third, the top half of the head, eyes, forehead, upper ear. Squeezing tightly in each position can cause different pain and results. For example, unless the legs are around the throat/neck a knockout probably won't ever happen. This can become a problem for girls with bigger legs and guys with shorter necks. In some cases the legs might not be able to squeeze the neck alone and might catch part of the jaw. This can hurt. This can hurt to the point where a knockout simply isn't possible because the male taps in agonizing pain before passing out. If the thighs are too big and cause excessive pain attempt a figure four position or calf based headscissors instead to get a knockout.

My advice, if avoiding pain or injury, is to never squeeze the jaw or lower half of the head alone. Obviously, some women have those man-mashing thighs larger than their loving victim's entire head. In those cases, the whole head probably will get squeezed, and if going for the neck some jaw pain may be guaranteed. If you are going for knock outs aim for the neck and neck alone. If you are going for headscissors without knockouts or just low pain aim for the eye level and above. The top half of the head can be squeezed harder and longer than the neck or jaw, but that still doesn't mean it should be squeezed with full might. It is a great idea to use proper communication and try the different positions with this placement in mind.

The worst type of headscissors, abusive headscissors. I'm not talking about abusive headscissors that were asked for. This is the literal use of headscissors to control and manipulate a partner outside of the bedroom against their will. While it may be rare, it can happen. Personally, like I've said before, if my partner were to headscissor me so she could get her way over something trivial like the restaurant we choose, I'd love it on an infrequent occasion. Regardless of my own desires, I advise against this because that is where abuse starts. It starts as a trivial thing that sometimes nobody even cares about. Then it becomes more frequent and over more important things. The best way to stop abuse is to prevent it. Keep headscissoring consensual and for pleasure or closeness, not for personal gain at the expense of the other partner. Does this mean you can't have your fantasy of being forced to go shopping with your girlfriend because she headscissored you until you agreed? Absolutely not! *Communicate* your desire for that in a healthy way. Can that lead to abusive behavior in the future? Perhaps, but this is your world. Be conscious of the risks before agreeing or asking to do anything.

If the abuse is, unfortunately, already present and not going anywhere anytime soon. I can't help you. I don't know enough about domestic abuse to confidently give you an answer. I can try, but in all reality it will likely end up hurting you more instead. I can, however, give you something that may be better suited for your needs. Here is a link to a website which organized a list of buyable books about this exact topic (not headscissor abuse but domestic abuse). While the first link is mostly catered towards women's domestic needs, which is fine, if experiencing serious headscissor abuse chances are you are a man at the mercy of a woman. I have found a website which contains books for men experiencing domestic abuse. I will write the link to it below the first link.

For women:

https://www.domesticshelters.org/resources/books/identifying-and-escaping-abuse

For men:

https://www.goodreads.com/list/show/155806.Domestic_Abuse_With_Male_Victims

Next I would like to quote an article which goes over sexual safety. It is about aftercare, an often overlooked aspect of sex that I highly recommend adding to the dynamic. A link will be provided if you are interested in reading the whole article.

"Aftercare is a post-play check-in, where partners give time and attention to each other to wrap up the scene and make sure everyone is feeling safe and comfortable. It can include cuddling, discussing the scene, drinking water, eating a snack, or something else. There aren't rules for what you "have" to do for aftercare because everyone is different, but the end goal should be to communicate and make sure everyone is feeling good and taken care of. Aftercare is for everyone involved in play, not just for the submissive partner(s). Dominant folks need aftercare too, so make sure to check in with everyone involved in a scene and see what they need for support."

Aftercare in the headscissoring sense can happen frequently or sparsely. The woman can stop to kiss the man and ensure he is doing just fine after literally every squeeze, every knock out, or once at the end of the session. It is all up to the parties at play, but some form of aftercare is highly recommended. Like the article said, aftercare isn't just for the man, but with the nature of headscissors the man might need a bit more aftercare and time to recover before attending to the woman's aftercare.

Before I get into the tips and advice for the different degrees, I want to quickly go over some things to avoid when it comes to headscissors.

Firstly, I advise avoiding anything both partners are not deeply consensual with. This can cause unnecessary stress and resentment, but the good thing is that with time and practice both parties can become comfortable or grow to want different things. Next, don't sleep in a headscissor. Don't go to bed for the night in a headscissor. The woman will fall asleep and not know if you're slowly dying from the pressure, and if you need to escape you'd have to muscle your way out since she's asleep. Does it sound fun and bond creating? Hell yeah! Have I attempted it? Well…I still must say, do it at your own risk if you do it at all.

Never start a session without properly communicating prior. That's a no brainer. Enough said. Then we have the super squeeze, or more commonly known as simply squeezing after a knock out. Can you do it? Yeah. Should you? Probably not. Is squeezing tightly five seconds after the man passes out going to kill him? No. Is squeezing tightly for sixty seconds after the man passes out going to kill him? Probably not, but he might throw up all over the place as his body attempts to wake him up for oxygen.

Don't headscissor in front of children. I don't even need to say anything else. Another thing to avoid is eating a heavy meal before a session. I can't explain the science behind it, but my guess is the heat, increased heart rate, changes in blood pressure, lack of oxygen, and flailing of the body might cause some nausea which is dangerous on a full stomach. Keep in mind if super squeezing after a knock out, the body can and will vomit in attempts to awaken itself. Lastly, do not think too hard about all the possible things not to do in a headscissor session. Especially as a man, for if you think of it there is a chance you may want to try it. This can be a blessing and a curse. Think away at your own risk!

## Tips and Advice for the Degrees

First up we have the soft headscissors, the **first four degrees** (1, 2, 3, 4). I grouped them together because they are quite similar and low risk. Remember, in the first degree the only requirement is that the woman's legs are around the male's head or body. They don't even have to be touching. In the fourth degree, physical contact, inability to escape, and soft squeezes or fast pulsing squeezes that do not force the male to tap out all occur.

My advice? Take it slow. There is no risk of getting knocked out or even tapping out. Enjoy the closeness you and your partner get to have together, and enjoy the soft squeezing that may temporarily stop your airflow or blood flow. For the women applying the hold, just keep him in tight. Not breath-squelching tight, but just tight enough that as much of your legs touch him as possible and escape is not an option. Remind him who is in charge by giving him the occasional tight squeeze for a few seconds or hit him with a combo of rapid-fire soft squeezes that are more so you literally flexing your muscles on him. If the position allows it, feel free to jiggle what your mother gave you in his face, and if you feel like it, smother him with whatever you want. Then proceed to squeeze or pulse your muscles occasionally. Put your legs around his upper head to avoid the most pain, and simply enjoy the fact that you have a man trapped between your legs! Enjoy the strength and power you have over him. If you are the man, bathe in the glory of her leg strength as she kindly shows you mercy between them.

A **fifth degree** headscissor session! Oh no, you're in trouble! In all actuality, not much changes here. The woman can aim for any placement around her man's head like before, but since tap outs are a staple of this degree more intense squeezing and action occurs. It can be in any position. To start out, squeeze as softly as you can and ever so gently squeeze harder until he taps. When the man taps, oblige. Release the pressure and drop it all the way down to a first degree headscissor where your legs aren't even touching him. Then after a few seconds rev up the man-mashers again, just as slowly as before. If you are the male start it off by being as weak as possible (assuming this is your first headscissor session for both man and woman). The second you start to feel pain, tap. Then when she squeezes again, tap a second after you feel the pain. Then two seconds. Then three. And so forth. Become accustomed to her leg strength in each position while she becomes accustomed to her own strength. Remember that she possesses the power to spice things up and grip you tight suddenly. As her victim, try to hold out until you start getting dizzy or can't handle the pain. The difference between a sixth degree and fifth degree headscissor can boil down to you trying your hardest just to resist her strength for even one more second. If you can't handle it, submit. She will love you even more knowing your own limits. She will adjust accordingly and quickly learn just how much of her you can handle, if any. That of course, is assuming you both wanted to take things slowly. Quick taps are also fair game in the fifth degree.

Things are getting serious. **Sixth degree** means a knockout is imminent, and if this is your first time things will be scary. Mentioned before, if trying a knockout for the first time please do it in a front facing headscissor. The woman needs to coil her thighs around the man's neck on each side, shoot them outwards, and lock the ankles. The man should be facing her crotch or stomach. He then should hold his hands upwards in the air while he awaits his demise. This way, since it is also the first time for her, she can see what it looks like when her thighs finish her victim. Immediately after his hands fall at all (they may not always fall), release the hold and make sure he is okay. It doesn't have to be in the same session, but my advice is to follow this method a handful of times until the woman is confident in her ability to notice when he has been knocked out. Please note that the falling of the hands may not always happen the instant the male falls unconscious.

Another, better option is the timed knockout. Slowly increasing the squeeze time is a safer alternative. If the male isn't knocked out after fifteen seconds of non-stop squeezing, upping the squeeze time to twenty means at the worst he is squeezed four seconds after he passes out. The time can be upped continuously until a knockout occurs, and the female will know when a knockout occurs because of the grace period where she communicates verbally to ensure consciousness. Between squeezes she will give the man time to communicate whether or not he fell unconscious. In my opinion, this method is the best for practicing knockouts, especially since it can be utilized in any position, including the reverse headscissor.

Assuming you and your partner have followed the instructions in the previous paragraph, a hard headscissor shouldn't be too difficult. This includes **degrees seven through nine** (7, 8, 9). Although, I wholeheartedly advise NEVER going to an eighth degree or higher. The main change between six and seven of course being two knockouts in one session. Eight is defined by lack of safety concern, visible and extreme pain, and holding a squeeze long after any knockouts, but let's focus on the seventh degree first. By now the woman SHOULD be confident and attentive when it comes to noticing when her partner is out cold. My tips here are simple. Aim for the neck. The more thigh you can fit on the neck the faster the knockout. Figure four's and their variants are great for knockouts, but I, and my biased opinion, recommend the reverse headscissor for this degree. The math is simple. Left thigh cradles one side of the neck. Right thigh cradles the other side of the neck. Asscheeks eat up the entire front portion of the neck. When they all team up and squeeze together at full strength…five seconds. That is the longest I'd last. That is also probably the longest you'd last. Full strength shouldn't even be required. The victim will still be out within thirty seconds even at half strength from the positioning alone. Once out, smack his face around until consciousness is back. Then, since we are hard headscissoring now, give a sly and flirtatious remark about how your ass put him to sleep before doing it all over again.

If the eighth degree is something you're looking for, aim for the jaw or squeeze at full strength until his nose bleeds. Safety is no longer a concern at the eighth degree. Get reckless. Tips for the man? Good luck. Taps can be ignored here. Consciousness can be taken. Your soul is hers. You will beg her for mercy at some point. You wanted the ticket, and you got it! Enjoy the ride!

# Chapter 10

## Finishing Up

So there you have it! I'll make it short and sweet. While this isn't everything there possibly is to learn about the sexual desire that is headscissoring, I hope this helped you with at least one question you had about headscissoring. Notice, not once did I ever refer to headscissoring as a kink or fetish instead of desire or need. There is nothing wrong with having a kink or a fetish, and headscissoring certainly can fall into those categories. The negative connotation surrounding those words might make some of you feel less about yourself since you enjoy this. Headscissoring for most, in all honesty, is a kink. If you enjoy it, then don't feel bad. Don't feel ashamed since you enjoy it when women squeeze you with their legs. Don't feel like you are less of a person for enjoying a submissive role, regardless of your gender. If you've read this far then chances are you or your partner likes to headscissor. This is **_OKAY_**. You have this kink. They have this kink. It is just another link in the chain. It may be the first and most important link at the very start of your chain, or it may be a link a few links down the chain that gets overlooked. Regardless, it is what makes your chain unique, that chain being your sexuality.

Whether you agree with anything I said at all in this book or not, thank you for taking the time to explore and learn more about yourself or your partner. This book pales in comparison to the vast community of headscissoring which exists and includes everyone from session girls posting online to the seemingly normal couple down the street that headscissor unbeknown to anyone else in the privacy of their home. Now you have a final decision to make. Are you or are you not going to be a part of this community?

# Sacred Scissor Time

Alone they are in a dim-lit room,
Two souls, like stars, amid the gloom.
Though distant now, they soon will find
Their souls merging, intertwined.

Headscissoring, an intimate art,
A journey from worlds apart.
Drawn by love's invisible thread,
She lures him into the bed.

As he draws near, the air ignites,
She promises things get tight.
Legs reach out, tentative and slow,
Eager for the intimacy to grow.

Quickly they coiled, his end now near,
She gains confidence from his visible fear.
Yet in her thigh's tender, soft embrace,
She provides a tranquil and harmless space.

Breathless whispers, skin to skin,
His passion burns, a flame within.
In this union, their souls align,
Bound by love, in sweet design.

She revels at his failed escapes,
Her taunting whispers, love is great.
He cherishes moments spent this way,
In between her legs all day he'd stay.

Large in charge, she feels his writhing soul,
But with every pulse, her heart can't control.
When he's between her legs, she breathes delight,
She'll find herself content, trapping the love of her life.

To her loving grip, he now slowly yields,
Once caught, his fate long ago was sealed.
Drifting off trapped by her thighs,
All his worries had quickly died.

So let them linger in this tender dance,
Lost in the magic of romance.
Headscissoring, an experience divine,
Where love's embrace, inescapable by design.

# Sources

## Chapter 2:

Crurophilia: https://www.yourdictionary.com/crurophilia

Femdom: https://www.yourdictionary.com/femdom

Humiliation Kink (Erotic Humiliation):
https://en.wikipedia.org/wiki/Erotic_humiliation

Masochism: https://www.merriam-webster.com/dictionary/masochism

Sadism: https://www.merriam-webster.com/dictionary/sadism

Male Opinions:
https://www.reddit.com/r/headscissors/comments/1afzxxo/why_headscisso rs/?force_seo=1

Female Opinions:
https://www.reddit.com/r/headscissors/comments/1at9nk3/why_headscisso r_ladies/

## Chapter 4:

Different takes on porn consumption if you are curious:

https://fightthenewdrug.org/10-reasons-why-porn-is-unhealthy-for-consum ers-and-society/

https://theconversation.com/is-watching-porn-bad-for-your-health-we-asked-5-experts-140550

https://metro.co.uk/2015/11/24/6-reasons-why-your-porn-habit-might-actually-be-good-for-you-5522338/

# Chapter 9:

Sources for additional kink safety:

Aftercare quote:
https://www.gstherapycenter.com/blog/2019/3/8/kink-safety-what-you-need-to-know

Femdom Guide:
https://themendingmuse.com/personal-growth/femdom-dominatrix/

Carotid Choking:
https://jerkmagazine.net/9mfehhs6kt2vag7aqn19w0hd2b5dka/safe-choking-101#:~:text=In%20order%20to%20properly%20choke,the%20ear%20than%20the%20chin.

Carotid Case Brazilian Jiu Jitsu:
https://www.ncbi.nlm.nih.gov/pmc/articles/PMC10621583/

Safe Choking: https://qcnerve.com/savage-love-safe-sexual-choking/

Kink Safety:
https://www.cosmopolitan.com/uk/love-sex/sex/a44876608/how-to-explore-kink-safely/

# Chapter 10:

Kink: https://en.wikipedia.org/wiki/Kink_(sexuality)

Fetish: https://en.wikipedia.org/wiki/Sexual_fetishism

Difference between fetish and kink:
https://www.masterclass.com/articles/kink-vs-fetish

# Special Thanks

I want to give a special thank you to Reddit user ElectricSqueeeze for providing the legs used in the cover of this book. The pose perfectly illustrates headscissoring as a whole even without the watermelon added.

I also want to thank the headscissoring community as a whole. All the enjoyers, fans, content creators, session girls, and anyone who has ever wanted, got caught in, or provided headscissors in a consensual environment, you deserve a round of applause and loads of respect. If it weren't for you, I may not have ever unearthed this sexual desire nor made this book. You all are the reason this community exists. Thank you for letting me be a part of it! And thank YOU, the reader, for taking the time to learn more about this beautiful art.

# About the Author:

Hello! I am the author of this incredibly strange book. Whether you use this as a guide book, how-to book, or informational book about headscissors, I made it because I myself enjoy headscissors. I couldn't say no to receiving one if my partner's intentions behind it were love fueled, and I wanted to learn more about this topic while also educating others. Instead of simply continuing to watch headscissor content, I decided to transmute that sexual energy into something tangible and helpful for the world! It just so happens to be a book mainly about girls headscissoring guys. By writing this I am attempting to give back to the world in a positive way. In doing so my goal is to help the headscissoring community better understand themselves or their sexual desires. Also, I wanted to promote this sexual desire in a positive and shame free manner. If this book manages to help even one person then I will consider it a successful endeavor.

www.ingramcontent.com/pod-product-compliance
Lightning Source LLC
Chambersburg PA
CBHW081647270326
41933CB00018B/3380